PTCE
The Ultimate Study Guide

Pass the Pharmacy Technician Certification Examination

Preface

This book will increase your chances of passing the PTCE. It will provide a review of the major topics in pharmacy with sample questions that will help you retain and assimilate more the information presented.

In addition, the answers to the sample questions are explained, so that you can learn from the answers, as well.

Have fun while learning.

© Copyright 2017 by Barfield All rights reserved.

This document is geared towards providing exact and reliable information in regards to the topic and issue covered. The publication is sold with the idea that the publisher is not required to render accounting, officially permitted, or otherwise, qualified services. If advice is necessary, legal or professional, a practiced individual in the profession should be ordered.

- From a Declaration of Principles which was accepted and approved equally by a Committee of the American Bar Association and a Committee of Publishers and Associations.

In no way is it legal to reproduce, duplicate, or transmit any part of this document in either electronic means or in printed format. Recording of this publication is strictly prohibited and any storage of this document is not allowed unless with written permission from the publisher. All rights reserved.

The information provided herein is stated to be truthful and consistent, in that any liability, in terms of inattention or otherwise, by any usage or abuse of any policies, processes, or directions contained within is the solitary and utter responsibility of the recipient reader. Under no circumstances will any legal responsibility or blame be held against the publisher for any reparation, damages, or monetary loss due to the information herein, either directly or indirectly.

Respective authors own all copyrights not held by the publisher.

The information herein is offered for informational purposes solely, and is universal as so. The presentation of the information is without contract or any type of guarantee assurance.

The trademarks that are used are without any consent, and the publication of the trademark is without permission or backing by the trademark owner. All trademarks and brands within this book are for clarifying purposes only and are the owned by the owners themselves, not affiliated with this document.

Table of content

Preface 2
Chapter 1: All about the PTC Exam 5
Chapter 2: How to Prepare for the PTC Exam 7
Chapter 3: Math and Calculations in Pharmacy 11
Chapter 4: Review Questions on Math and Calculations 42
Chapter 5: Answers to Review Questions in Math and Calculations
.... 47
Chapter 6: Most Significant Conversion Factors 65
Chapter 7: Review Questions on Conversion Factors 69
Chapter 8: Answers to Quiz on Conversion Factors 70
Chapter 9: SI Units of Measurements.. 76
Chapter 10: Statistics in Pharmacy 78
Chapter 11: Important Medical Transcriptions and Abbreviations .85
Chapter 12: Arabic and Roman numerals....................................... 91
Chapter 13: Review Questions on Statistics and Numerals 94
Chapter 14: Answers to the Review Questions 97
Chapter 15: Common Drugs You Must Know............................... 102
Chapter 16: Pointers in Assisting the Pharmacist in Serving Patients
.... 108
Chapter 17: Inventory Control Systems 115
Chapter 18: System of Maintaining Medication Quality............... 117
Chapter 19: Administration and Management of Pharmacy Practice
.... 120
Chapter 20: Responsibilities of a Pharmacy Technician to Patients
.... 124
Chapter 21: Review Questions for the PTC Exams 128
Chapter 22: Answers to Review Questions on PTC Exams.......... 136
Conclusion 153

Chapter 1: All about the PTC Exam

The PTC exam is the Pharmacy Technician Certification Board examination, which is responsible in rendering the PTCE, the Pharmacy Technician Certification Exam.

What is the purpose of the PTC exam?

This examination is conducted to test the knowledge and abilities of Pharmacy Technicians who want to seek national accreditation for their profession. Once the examinee passed this exam, they will be able to obtain their credentials as a Certified Pharmacy Technician (CPT).

The CPT will increase the Pharmacy Technician's credibility, which will help him gain employment more easily.

What topics comprise the PTC exam?

There are three (3) major topics that are included. These are:

1. Assisting the pharmacist in serving patients
2. Maintaining medication and inventory control systems
3. Management and administration of pharmacy practice

The length of time of the exam is 2 hours.

Total number of items = 90 items (10 unscored, which is randomly distributed in the questionnaire, and 80 scored items)

Type of questions – multiple type questions with 4 choices of answers.

What are the requirements for the PTCE certification?

1. High school diploma or equivalent GED diploma
2. No criminal records
3. No violations of the pharmacy code of conduct
4. Passing score in the PTCE (Pharmacy Technician Certification Exam)
5. Compliance and non-violation with/of PTCE certification policies

Chapter 2: How to Prepare for the PTC Exam

As pharmacy technicians, it's natural that you aspire for a certification. This will assure you of a more fruitful career in the future.

So, how can you prepare for the PTC exam?

Step #1 – Prepare yourself mentally

The first step is to be positive. It's not rocket science that every endeavor you venture on will require your dedication and an optimistic attitude.

Have you ever heard of the cliché, "If you think you can, you can"? Yesiree! You can do what you have set your mind to do because the mind is a powerful tool - if harnessed correctly.

You must possess this positive attitude while you prepare for the exam and during the exam itself. This good behavior will boost your performance in the test.

Step #2 – Prepare a timetable together with the corresponding goals

Prepare your review timetable, and opposite it, you write down your goals for that particular time. Be sure that your timetable is in congruence with the date you have set for your PTC Exam.

See table below:

Time allotted	Math, Calculations	Assisting the Pharmacy in delivering	Administration and Management of

		Services	pharmacy
1st week Feb 1 – Feb 8	At the end of the 1st week, I would have finished reviewing half of the review material (you can be more specific here by identifying the specific topics)	At the end of the 1st week, I would have reviewed half of the sub-topics	At the end of the 1st week, I would have finished reviewing half of the sub-topics.
2nd week Feb 9- Feb 16	At the end of the 2nd week, I would have finished reviewing the last half of the review materials	At the end of 2nd week, I would have finished reviewing the last half of the review material	At the end of 2nd week, I would have finished reviewing the last half of the review material
3rd week	At the end of the 3rd week, I would have passed the mock exams about this topic.	At the end of the 3rd week, I would have passed the mock exams about this topic.	At the end of the 3rd week, I would have passed the mock exams about this topic.

Step #3 - Gather relevant resources

Gather your review materials. Don't rely on old books solely. Search for updated review books. You can also utilize online resources.

Step #3 – Implement your timetable

Follow your schedule religiously. It's recommended to go to a library. This will discourage you from sleeping. You can take short breaks but stick to your timetable.

Step #4 – Before the night of the exam, sleep early

Cramming is not advisable because this will stress you out and you may be sleepy during the exam itself. That's why your review timetable must provide you ample time to rest and relax before the actual exam.

Step #5 – Before the exams, eat a hearty meal

The food of your neurons or brain cells is glucose and glucose comes from food (carbohydrates). You have to eat properly to boost the performance of your brain cells. You won't be able to think on an empty stomach. Don't gorge yourself, however, because this could also give you indigestion.

Step #6 - Attend to the call of nature before the exams

Never go to the exam venue if you have not emptied your bladder or your bowel. There are reported cases of failure because of the inability of the examinee to continue due to this reason.

Step #7 – Double check that you have brought all your materials with you

The PTC exam is computer based, so ascertain that you have what you need. The exam is conducted within 2 hours. Be prepared to stay that long in the testing sites.

What to do during the exams

Step #1 – Listen to the instructions carefully

Don't start answering, unless you have understood the instructions fully.

Step #2 - Read the questions, at least twice, before answering

Don't skip any question. If you don't know the answer, analyze the question and make an educated guess.

Step #3 – Take note of the time

You can practice beforehand how long 2 hours is based on your perception. This way you can have a 'feel' of its length.

Step #4 – Relax while taking the test

Anxiety may cause 'temporary amnesia'. Avoid stressing yourself. The worst thing that could happen to you is that you fail. Nevertheless, it's not the end of the world. Thus, just enjoy your time answering the questions.

With a positive mind, ample preparation and a relax mind and body, there's no reason you won't pass the exams.

Chapter 3: Math and Calculations in Pharmacy

In pharmacy, you need to know your math and calculations because you need to compute every now and then in preparing your solutions or medications.

Here are some practice problems that can help you with your computations during the PTC exams.

DILUTIONS

Dilutions are required when you have to prepare a weaker solution from a stronger solution.

Take note that when you dilute substances, the resulting solution would be less concentrated because you have added a diluent.

Your diluent can be distilled water, normal saline solution or other preparations that may be needed by the procedure.

Here are examples:

Let's say the instruction is to prepare a 1:10 dilution of the stock solution, and the recommended diluent is distilled water.

The first thing to remember is that 1:10 means that 1 part of the diluent is added to 9 parts of the solute to produce a 1:10 dilution.

Thus:

1 part solute + 9 parts diluent = 10 parts, hence dilution is 1:10

The easiest method to prepare is to equate 1 part to 1 mL (milliliters) and 9 parts to 9 mL or ml.

Hence:

1 ml solute + 9 ml diluent will give a 1:10 dilution.

The problem, however, is that sometimes the volume of solute may not be as much as 1 ml. What can you do if you encounter this problem?

It's easy, just consider the available volume of your solute as 1 part.

Example #1:

If the available volume of your solute is 0.5 ml, you equate this to 1 part.

Now, your next problem would be, how many ml of diluent will you be adding?

This problem is easy too, all you have to do is to determine the volume of diluent that is equivalent to 9 parts, if 1 part is equal to 0.5 ml.

How do you do that?

Just multiply 0.5 ml (1 part) with 9 (parts).

So, 0.5 ml x 9 = 4.5 ml

Hence to prepare a 1:10 dilution when your solute is 0.5 ml, you simply add 0.5 ml of the solute to 4.5 ml o the diluent. This will give a 1:10 dilution.

Example #2:

How can you prepare a 1:5 dilution?

Use the easiest method, consider 1 part as 1 ml.

Hence:

To prepare a 1:5 dilution of solution, add 1 ml of solute to 4 ml of solvent or diluent.

If you have noticed, the last number after the colon is the sum of the parts of the solute and the solvent (diluent). In this instance the solute must be in the liquid form.

If the solute is in the solid form, you have to convert it first to a liquid form. This will be discussed later on.

What about if the available solute is only 0.2 ml?

Consider 0.2 ml as 1 part.

Thus:

0.2 ml of solute + 0.8 ml of diluent (0.2 x 4) = 1:5 dilution of solution

      1 part   +   4 parts = 5 parts - 1:5 dilution

What about if the total volume is given?

Example #3:

How can you prepare a 1:10 dilution with a total volume of 18 ml?

You have to consider 18 ml as the total volume. Therefore, if 18 ml is 10 parts, how can you get the volume of the solute and the diluent?

You have to divide 18 by 10.

18/10 = 1.8

Hence, your 1 part would be 1.8 ml and your 9 parts would be 16.2 ml (9 x 1.8).

So, you add 1.8 ml of solute to 16.2 ml of solvent to prepare a 1:10 diluted solution.

1.8 ml (1 part) + 6.2 ml (9 parts) = 18 ml

1 part + 9 parts = 10 parts; 1:10 dilution.

SERIAL DILUTIONS

This is a systematic re-dilution of solutions. It's often used in preparing varying concentrations of the drug. It has various uses, such as in case studies of drug medications, in preparing weaker drug concentrations, and in preparing working solutions.

Example #1:

The doctor requested that the pharmacist test different concentrations of the drug, using a serial dilution.

The pharmacist prepared three test tubes (tt).

To all tubes, he added 1 ml of the diluent.

Then to the first tube, he added 0.50 ml of the solute.

14

He mixed the solution thoroughly and then pipetted 0.5 ml of this solution and added it to test tube 2.

He mixed this solution in tube 2 and pipetted 0.5 ml of this solution to the 3rd tube.

He mixed it anew and then pipetted 0.5 ml and discarded it.

Question: What are the final dilutions of each tube?

Tabulating the given data will give you a clearer view of what the given data and unknown are:

	test tube 1	test tube 2	test tube 3
Volume of solute	0.50 ml	0.50 ml from tt1	0.50 ml from tt2
Volume of solvent (diluent)	1 ml	1 ml	1 ml
Dilution of tube itself	1:3	1:3	1:3
Final dilution	1:3	1:9 (1:3 x 1:3)	1:27 (1:9 x 1:3)

The dilution 1:3 is obtained by solving the dilution from the given data:

 Volume of solute = 0.5 ml = 1 part

 Volume of solvent = 1 ml = 2 parts (based on 0.5 ml as 1 part)

 1 part (solute) + 2 parts (solvent) = 3 parts

 Thus, dilution is 1:3 for each of the tube itself.

The second tube has a different computation because of the diluted solute that is used, you have to multiple the dilution of the tube itself with the dilution of the previous tube (1:3) to get 1:9

For tube 3, you have to multiply the dilution of the tube itself, 1:3, with the dilution of the previous tube from where you obtained the diluted solute.

1:3 x 1:9 = 1:27

You could easily solve the final dilution by remembering the following pointers:

- Dilution does NOT always represent the volume.
- Dilution is the sum of the PARTS of the solute and the solvent. (the part of the solute, which is typically 1 part + the parts of the diluent or solvent).
- In serial dilutions, remember to multiply the dilution of the previous tube, from where you got the diluted solute, with the dilution of the tube itself. (See examples above.)
- Consider the total volume in the computations, if this is given in the problem.

RATIOS

Ratio is different from dilutions. In dilutions, the solute and solvent (diluent) parts are added, while in ratios, they remain as is.

Example #1:

When we say the ratio of the solution is 1:10, we are actually saying that 1 part of the solute is added to 10 parts of the solvent.

Hence, the volume will be:

1 ml solute + 10 ml solvent or diluent

Of course, if you get the dilution of this same solution, the dilution would be 1:11 (1 part solute + 10 parts solvent = 11 parts, thus the dilution is 1:11.

Example #2:

If you are asked to prepare a 1: 18 ratio of solution, you will have to prepare it this way:

1 part solute + 18 parts solvent

Again, if you get the dilution of this same solution, it would be: 1:19 dilution.

Therefore:

In ratios, you don't add the solute and solvent parts, while in dilutions, you add the solute and solvent parts to obtain the resulting dilution.

RATIO and PROPORTION

Ratio and proportion is often used to solve for patient dosages. It's also one of the methods that you can use for other computations.

The first thing that you must remember is that the units of the numerators must be the same, likewise with your denominators.

If they are not, then you have to convert them to similar units first, before you can solve your math equation. Make sure that they are referring to the same item, as well.

If the first volume is in milliliters and the second volume is in liters, you can either convert the volumes to milliliters or vice versa. It's up to you. Just ascertain that they are in similar units.

Example #1:

You are tasked to prepare a 150 ml of 75% working solution from a 95% stock solution.

In this problem, you have to know the volume of solute and solvent to be able to prepare the 75% working solution.

Using ratio and proportion, you can do it this way:

150 ml/75% = X/95%

Or

$$\frac{150 \text{ ml}}{75\%} = \frac{X}{95\%}$$

Cross multiply the equations:

150 ml x 75% = X x 95%

Then isolate (cancel out) X by transposing 95% from the right equation by dividing both equations by 95%.

$$\frac{150 \text{ ml} \times 75\%}{} = \frac{X \times 95\%}{}$$

$$\frac{150 \text{ ml} \times 75\%}{95\%} = X$$

$$118.4210 \text{ ml} = X$$

or X = 118.4 ml of 95% of stock solution

The percent signs are canceled out, and the ml sign is carried out. Therefore, when you solve the problem, the answer is 118.4 ml. This is the volume of the solute or the 95% stock solution that you need to prepare your working solution. But, you have to solve the volume of your diluent or solvent too.

Since the final volume is 150 ml, you can solve for the volume of the diluent by subtracting the volume of the solute from your total volume. The solute is the smaller volume between the two substances.

Thus:

$$150 - 118.4 = 31.6 \text{ ml of diluent or solvent}$$

You can now prepare your 150-ml working solution by adding 118.4 ml of 95% stock solution to 31.6 ml diluent or solvent.

Example #2

What dosage will you give a patient weighing 45 pounds, if your basis is 250 milligrams for a 120-pound patient.

Using ratio and proportion, you can create your computation this way:

250 mg : 120 pounds = X (mg) : 45 pounds

Cross multiply:

250 x 45 = 120 x X

Cancel 120 mg from the right equation, or transpose to isolate X, through division:

$$\frac{250 \times 45}{120} = \frac{120 \times X}{120}$$

$$X = \frac{250 \times 45}{120}$$

X = 93.75 mg – dosage for a 45-pound patient.

Example #3

You have an instruction from the attending physician to give 500 mg of the therapeutic drug to your patient. If 6 ml is equal to 0.50 grams (g), who many ml would you give the patient?

You can also use ratio and proportion in this problem. But before you can do it, convert the units to like units first. Since milligrams is the more common unit in drug dosages, you can choose to change the grams to milligrams. Take note that either way is correct.

In this particular problem, we will opt to convert the grams to milligrams. Since 1,000 mg is equal to 1 gram, using ratio and proportion, you can use it this way:

Step #1 – Convert units to similar units.

$$\frac{1,000 \text{ mg}}{1 \text{ gram}} = \frac{X \text{ (mg)}}{0.50 \text{ grams}}$$

or 1,000: 1 = x:0.50

Cross multiply:

1,000 mg x 0.50 grams = X x 1 gram

Again, to cancel 1 gram from the right equation, divide it by 1 gram. Whatever you do to the right equation, you should also do this to the left equation.

$$\frac{1,000 \text{ mg} \times 0.50 \text{ gram}}{1 \text{ grams}} = \frac{X \times 1 \text{ gram}}{1 \text{ grams}}$$

The 'grams' unit will be canceled out. Solving the equation, you will come up with the answer.

X = *500 mg is equivalent to 0.50 grams*

Step #2 – Solve for the ml of the dosage

Now, you have similar units, you can now use ratio and proportion to solve for the ml of the dosage:

6 ml: 500 mg = X (ml):500 mg

Cross multiply:

6 ml x 500 mg = 500 mg x X(ml)

Cancel out or transpose 500 mg (see above, for more explanations).

$$\frac{6 \text{ ml} \times 500 \text{ mg}}{500 \text{ mg}} = \frac{500 \text{ mg} \times X(\text{ml})}{500 \text{ mg}}$$

Solving the equation, your answer would be:

X = 6 ml dosage

In this particular case, just by analyzing the problem, you know immediately that the answer is 6 because it has been given already.

In summary, you can solve the volume in ml of the dosage, through this formula:

$$\text{Unknown} = \frac{\text{Doctor's order} \times \text{volume of drug available}}{\text{Dose on hand}}$$

You can apply this formula to the problem above:

$$\text{Required dosage in ml} = \frac{500 \text{ mg} \times 6 \text{ ml}}{500 \text{ mg}}$$

Answer = 6 ml

PERCENT SOLUTIONS

When computing the percentage of anything the general formula is:

$$\% = \frac{\text{number of specific values} \times 100}{\text{Total number of values}}$$

Example:

If you want to compute for the percentage of PTCE passers, wherein 2,355 passed out of 6,350, you can use the general formula:

$$\% = \frac{\text{number of specific values} \times 100}{\text{Total number of values}}$$

$\% = 2,355/6350 \times 100$

% = 0.3708661417322835 x 100

% = **37.08661417322835 %**

In the field of pharmacy, you will often compute for the percentages of the following solutions:

1. Weight/volume percent solutions
2. Weight/weight percent solutions
3. Volume/volume percent solutions

Weight/volume percent solutions

For the weight/volume percent solutions, the formula is:

% = W/V x 100

Where: W = weight of solute in grams

V = total volume of solution

Example #1:

You are tasked to prepare a 23%, weight over volume, sodium chloride (NaCl) solution. In this problem, you need to compute for the weight of solute (NaCl). Using the general formula of percentage given above, you can derive the formula for the weight in grams of solute.

$$\% = \frac{W \times 100}{V}$$

$$\% \times V = W \times 100$$

$$W = \frac{\% \times V}{100}$$

Substitute the values in the formula.

$$\text{Weight in grams of solute} = \frac{23 \times V}{100}$$

Since the total volume is not indicated, you can assume any volume that you need. The easiest is to assume that the total volume is 100 ml.

Thus:

$$\text{W in grams of solute} = \frac{23 \times 100}{100}$$

W = 23 grams (g) of NaCl is diluted with distilled water or diluent up to the 100-ml mark of a volumetric flask.

You have to keep in mind that you don't just add the 23 grams of sodium chloride powder to 100 ml of distilled water, because this will produce more than 100 ml solution, which will be inaccurate.

Your final volume must be exactly 100 ml. To ensure this, you have to make use of a volumetric flask in preparing the solution. The volumetric flask is the most accurate apparatus in preparing solutions.

There are two ways to prepare the 23% sodium chloride solution (NaCl).

First, you can add half of the total volume to the flask, then add 23 grams of NaCl powder. Mix until the powder is dissolved. Then, add the diluent up to the 100-ml mark. Ensure that you don't add more than the mark. You can use a dropper when the volume is nearing the 100-ml mark, so that you can safely stop at 100-ml mark.

The second method is to place the powder first in the volumetric flask, then add half of the total volume and dissolve the powder completely. Afterwards, add the diluent up to the 100-ml mark in the flask.

Weight /weight percent solutions

For w/w percent solutions, you can use the same formula, but this time both your solute and solvent are measured using their weight in grams.

Hence:

$$\% = \frac{\text{Weight in grams of solute} \times 100}{\text{Weight in grams of solution}}$$

Example:

You are tasked to prepare 18% calcium chloride ($CaCl_2$) solution, using w/w.

Since the weight in grams of solution is not indicated, you can assume that it is 100 grams.

Hence:

Solving for the weight in grams of solute, you have to cross-multiply the equation:

% x Weight in grams of solution = weight in grams of solute x 100

Transpose Weight in grams of solution to be able to solve the Weight in grams of solute: This is a simple math equation, so I know I don't have to elaborate. But just in case: to transpose, you have to remove 100 from the second equation by cancelling it out through division. However, whatever you do to the right equation, you should also do this to the left equation, thus:

$$\frac{\text{Weight in grams of solute} \times 100}{100} = \frac{\% \times \text{Weight in grams of solution}}{100}$$

The resulting formula would be:

$$\text{Weight in grams of solute} = \frac{\% \times \text{weight in grams of solution}}{100}$$

Substituting the given values in the formula, you will obtain:

$$\text{Weight in grams of solute} = \frac{18 \times 100}{100}$$

Weight in grams of solute = 18 grams of CaCl2

Since the units are the same or similar, you can simply weigh the 18 grams of CaCl2 and add it to 82 grams of solvent (weight of solvent = 100 grams – 18 grams of solute = 82 grams of solvent.)

Volume/volume percent solutions

You can use the same formula, but this time, you use volumes instead of weights.

Example:

$$\% = \frac{\text{Volume of solute} \times 100}{\text{Volume of solution}}$$

Cross-multiplying the equation will give you:

% x Volume of solution = Volume of solute x 100

Transpose Volume of solution to be able to solve the volume of solute:

$$\text{Volume of solute} = \frac{\% \times \text{volume of solution}}{100}$$

Example #1

How can you prepare a 20% solution (V/V) with a total volume of 120 ml?

$$\text{Volume of solute} = \frac{\% \times \text{volume of solution}}{100}$$

$$\text{Volume of solute} = \frac{20 \times 120}{100}$$

Volume of solute = 24 ml

Example #2:

How can you prepare 10% of Hydrochloric acid (HCl) with a total volume of 150 ml?

$$\text{Volume of solute} = \frac{10 \times 150}{}$$

Volume of solute = 15 ml of HCl acid

Since they have the same units (ml), you can simply measure and add them directly. The total volume of the solution is 150 ml. Subtract the volume of solute, to obtain the volume of the diluent.

Volume of diluent = total volume of solution − volume of solute

Volume of diluent = 150 − 15 = 135 ml

Therefore, to prepare a 10% of hydrochloric acid (HCl) with a total volume of 150 ml, you have to add 15 ml of hydrochloric acid to 135 ml of distilled water or diluent.

SPECIFIC GRAVITY

You may have to compute the specific gravity of solutions from time to time. Specific gravity is defined as the ratio of the weight or density of a substance in grams over the weight or density of an equal volume of water in grams.

The formula is:

Specific Gravity = <u>Weight or density of substance in grams</u>

Weight or density of an equal volume of water in grams

Example:

What is the specific gravity of a substance that weighs 50 grams and in 120 ml of diluent?

Sp. Gr. = 50/120

Sp. Gr. = 0.4166667

N.B.

The weight of 120 ml of diluent is 120 grams because the density of water AST (at specified temperature – usually 4 degrees centigrade - is 1.)

DECIMAL NUMBERS

Decimal numbers can be rounded off to whole numbers by adding one to the previous digit if the number is more than 5.

If the number is less than 5, then leave the previous number unchanged.

Example #1:

Round off 1.23673 to two digits.

Look at the third number, if it's more than 5 add 1 to the 2nd digit, if not leave the 2nd digit as is. Since the third digit number is 6, which is more than 5, you have to add 1 o the 2nd digit.

So, the answer is: 1.24

Example #2:

Round off 2.3019 to a whole number:

Answer: 2

This is because you start with 9 and cancel it out, and add 1 to the previous digit to make it 2, cancel out 2, then 0, and then 3 because they are all less than 5. That leaves the whole number 2.

FRACTIONS

You have learned solving fractions in your basic math. But let's have a simple review, anyhow.

If the denominators of the fractions are the same, then you can add all the numerators.

Example:

If you have these fractions with the same denominators (2/3, 3/3, 1/3), you can add them.

2/3 + 3/3 + 1/3 = 6/3

Also, you can divide the value to get a whole number:

6/3 = 2

You can also divide them first before adding:

2/3 = 0.666666666666667

3/3 = 1

1/3 = 0.3333333333333333

Add all the quotients and you will obtain the same answer = **2**

IV FLOW RATES

Knowing how to compute for IV Flow Rates is vital for your profession. The IV Flow Rate is the number of drops per minute, or milliliter per hour, or liter per hour that an intravenous fluid is administered to patients. The most common is number of drops per minute (gtt/min).

Keep in mind that there are several factors affecting the IV Flow Rates. These include the drop factors (length and diameter of the needle), the volume of the solution and the order of the doctor.

Example:

The doctor ordered that a 2,000 ml of intravenous fluid should be administered to the patient within 16 hours. The drop factor of the apparatus is 20 drops per ml. How many drops per minute should be the IV Flow Rate?

Formula:

IV Flow Rate in gtt/min = <u>Volume of fluid to be infused x drop factor</u>

                                  Allotted time in minutes

$$\text{IV Flow Rate in gtt/min} = \frac{2{,}000 \text{ ml} \times 20 \text{ gtt/ml}}{16 \times 60 \text{ (to obtain minutes)}}$$

$$= 40{,}000 \text{ gtt}/960 \text{ minutes}$$

$$= \mathbf{41.67 \text{ gtt/min} \text{ or } 42 \text{ gtt/min}}$$

CHEMOTHERAPY DOSAGES

There are various factors that can affect a drug entering the body, such as patient's body surface area (BSA), and the drug elimination capability of the patient's body (patient's metabolism, physiological functions).

In the use of cytotoxic drugs, under dosing and overdosing can happen easily. Under dosing can reduce the effectiveness of the drug, while overdosing is harmful to the patient because it increases cytotoxicity and may cause death.

Using the body surface area of the patient as the only basis of drug dosage has shown limitations. BSA is not as accurate as it was previously known. This is due to the unpredictability of various factors affecting the drug's transport and metabolism inside the body.

There are various formulas used in computing for the BSA in square meters. The most common is using the formula of DuBois and DuBois:

$$BSA = 0.007184 \times (\text{Weight in kg})^{0.425} \times (\text{Height in cm})^{0.725}$$

And the Mosteller formula:

$$BSA = 0.016667 \times Weight^{0.5} \times Height^{0.5}$$

Example:

A 30-year old, male patient has the following data:

Drug dosage per square meters = 100

Weight in kg = 6 kg

Height in cm = 55 cm

Solve for the BSA using the DuBois and DuBois:

$$BSA = 0.007184 \times (6\ kg)^{0.425} \times (55\ cm)^{0.725}$$

BSA = 0.28 m² (square meters)

You can use too, the Mosteller formula:

$$BSA = 0.016667 \times (6\ kg)^{0.5} \times (55\ cm)^{0.5}$$

BSA = 0.31 m² (square meters)

Aside from BSA, always use other parameters, such as drug elimination, patient's organ status as related to the disposition of the drug when it enters the system, GFR or Glomerular Filtration Rate, CYP450 or cytochrome P450, the gene family that can affect the metabolism of drugs, to determine the correct dosage.

Patients who have extreme values (obese weights) cannot use the formula. The BSA formula is considered inaccurate and is used primarily to establish the absolute range within typical patients.

Therapeutic Drug Monitoring (TDM) is one way of evaluating the sub-therapeutic, therapeutic and toxic dosage for the patient. It's individualized so drug treatment becomes individualized too.

HALF-LIFE

TDM will sometimes require you to measure the peaks and troughs of the drug through blood samples. You may also be asked to determine the half-life of a drug. The half-life is the amount of time that the concentration of a drug is reduced to half of its original concentration.

Example #1:

What is the half-life of a drug if it has an original concentration of 650 mg and was reduced to 300 after an hour?

The half-life concentration of the drug is 325 mg (650/2).

The given is that after 1 hour (60 minutes), there was a 350-mg reduction from the original concentration (650-300 = 350).

Hence, you can use ratio and proportion to determine the amount of time that the original concentration was reduced to 325 mg.

350 mg: 60 minutes = 325 mg: X

Cross multiply:

350 x X = 60 x 325 mg

Cancel out 350 from the left equation to isolate X, the unknown. (You can position too this equation on the right; as long as the values are correct. You can also place time (in minutes) as the numerator, provided the other numerator is also 'time' (in minutes).

Obviously, your units should also be alike for the numerators of both equations, and the units of the denominators of both equations are the same, as well. (Refer to earlier discussions on ratio and proportion.)

X = 60 minutes x 325 mg/350 mg

X = 55.71 minutes

The half-life of the drug is 55.71 minutes.

You could also compute by determining how many milligrams is the drug concentration reduced per minute. You can do this by dividing 350 mg/60 minutes.

Amount of drug reduced per minute = **350/60** = **5.83333333333333**

This means that every minute the drug is reduced by 5.8333 grams. Hence, to get the half-life of the drug, divide the half-life concentration with the amount of milligrams per minute.

Half-life = 325/5.83333333333333

Half-life = 55.71 minutes

You will be obtaining the same answer as the first computation that used the ratio and proportion method.

DOSAGES

In computing for patients' dosages, the role of pharmacokinetics and pharmacodynamics must not be discounted. This indicates that you must know how the drug interacts with the body system and how it is eliminated from the body.

The most common basis of dosages are the weights and the ages of the patients. There are established values that are products of previous researches, so you can use these for your ratio and proportion method. Review examples given above.

SOLUTIONS and CONCENTRATIONS

A solution is composed of a solute and solvent/diluent. The solute can be in powder or liquid form.

When both solute and solvent are in liquid form, the substance with the lesser volume is the solute.

The simplest formula to compute for the concentrations or volumes of solutions is to use the formula:

$C_1 V_1 = C_2 V_2$

Where:

C_1 = original concentration

V_1 = original volume

C_2 = final concentration

V_2 = final volume

The ratio and proportion can also be used in this problem. Ratio and proportion can be used in countless of math calculations provided that the given data is appropriate, and you know how to create your equations.

Example #1:

How can you prepare a 15% solution with a total volume (TV) of 120 ml from a 20% solution?

Using the formula, $C_1V_1 = C_2V_2$, you can substitute the values. But, analyze the given first.

C_1 = 20%

V_1 = unknown (X)

C_2 = 15%

V_2 = 120 ml

Thus:

20% x V_1 (ml) = 15% x 120 ml

V_1 = 15% x 120 ml/20%

The percent unit will cancel each other out and the ml units will remain.

$$V_1 = 90 \text{ ml}$$

Your computation does not stop there. You still have to solve for the volume of your diluent. Your total volume is 120 ml, and 90 ml is only your V_1.

Solve for the volume of the diluent by subtraction the V_1 (90 ml) from the total volume (TV), 120 ml.

Volume of diluent = 120 ml – 90 ml

Volume of diluent = 30 ml

Therefore, the answer is:

To prepare a 15% solution with a total volume of 120 ml, you have to add 90 ml of the 20% solution to 30 ml of diluent.

Example #2:

How can you prepare 20 ml of a 15-mg working solution from a stock solution of 20 mg?

$C_1V_1 = C_2V_2$

20 mg x V_1 = 15 mg x 20 ml

C_1 = 15 mg x 20 ml/20 mg

C_1 = 15 ml of the 20-mg solution

To prepare the solution, add 15 ml of the 20-mg solution to 5 ml of diluent to produce a 15-mg solution with a total volume of 20 ml.

During the exams, if you don't remember the formula for a particular computation, you can try using ratio and proportion.

Chapter 4: Review Questions on Math and Calculations

Let's see if you can answer these review questions on math and pharmacy calculations. Try not to look at the answers while solving the problems. There is only one correct answer, thus read the questions twice or thrice before finalizing your answers.

N.B. In the actual PTCE exams, the questions are multiple types. In these examples, however, you will have to give the correct answer yourself to many of the questions. This is to increase your understanding, retention, and analytical skills.

Many PTCE takers say that the math and computations are the most difficult portion of the exam. However, if you understand the problem correctly, solving it would be a breeze. Therefore, the first step for you is to determine carefully what the given are, and what the unknown is.

QUESTIONS

1. You are preparing working solutions to test a new therapeutic drug manufactured by your company. How can you prepare 30 ml of each of the following working solutions from a 30-mg stock solution?

Concentration of working solution	Volume of 30 mg stock solution	Volume of diluent	Resulting dilution
5 mg			
10 mg			

20 mg			

2. The attending physician of a 10-year old male patient has ordered that the patient's 250-ml IV fluid must be administered within 2 hours. The drop factor of the IV is 15 ml per drop. What would be the correct IV flow rate?

3. An out-patient has to take 1,500 mg of erythromycin in three divided doses per day, for a period of 1 week. If 250 mg is equal to 5 ml, how many ml will you dispense for the whole treatment?

4. How can you prepare a 50% solution of methanol with a total volume of 170 ml from a 95% methanol solution?

5. A drug with an original concentration of 800mg has been reduced to 200 mg after 90 minutes. What's the half-life of the drug?

6. What dosage (in ml) would you give a patient weighing 130 pounds (lbs.) if the standard dosage is 0.1 ml per 1 kilogram (kg)?

7. You have performed these serial dilutions, while preparing your experimental drugs:

	Test Tube 1	Test Tube 2	Test Tube 3	Test Tube 4
	Volume in milliliters	Volume in milliliters	Volume in milliliters	Volume in milliliters

Serum/diluted serum	0.75 of pure serum	0.75 from tube 1 after mixing with df	0.75 from tube 2 after mixing with df	0.75 from tube 3 after mixing with df. Discard 0.75 of the solution after mixing
Diluting fluid (df)	3	3	3	3
Final dilution				

What is the final dilution of test tube no. 4?

A. 1: 25

B. 1: 625

C. 1:3125

D. 1:125

E. 1:27

8. How can you prepare a 1:10 dilution?

A. In a test tube pipet 1 milliliter of serum and add 10 milliliters of diluent.

B. In a test tube pipet 0.5 milliliter of serum and add 4.5 milliliter of diluent.

C. In a test tube pipet 10 milliliters of serum and add 1 milliliter of diluent.

D. In a test tube pipet 0.9 milliliter of serum and add 10 milliliters of diluent.

E. In a test tube pipet 0.5 milliliter of serum and add 9.5 milliliter of diluent.

9. What is the dilution if you have added 0.25 milliliters of serum to 2 milliliters of normal saline solution?

   A. 0.25:2

   B. 1:9

   C. 2:0.25

   D. 1:8

   E. 1:2.25

10. A 13-year old girl suffering from nausea and vomiting was brought to the infirmary. The physician ordered 0.8 mg/kg to be injected stat. The girl weighed 120 pounds. If 1 ml is equivalent to 5 mg, how many ml would you dispense?

11. Express the concentration of the following substances in SI units:

    a) 120 mg/dL glucose value
    b) 3 feet
    c) 24 hours

12. The doctor ordered a tapering dosage of tranxene caps 5 mg, an anxiolytic drug, for a patient who has anxiety

disorders. How many tranxene capsules would you dispense, if these were the orders?
a) 30 mg/d. in divided doses x 3 d
b) 20 mg/d. in divided doses x 3 d
c) 15 mg/d. x 5 d
d) 10 mg/d x 10 d

13. A drug is supplied in 250 mg tablets. If the prescription order is 250 mg b.i.d for a period of 10 days, how many tablets would you dispense?

14. If you have dissolved 25 grams of substance in 160 ml of distilled water, what is the:
2.1. % (W/V)
2.2. Specific gravity

Chapter 5: Answers to Review Questions in Math and Calculations

Here are the correct answers to the review questions in chapter 4. For each of the questions, an explanation is provided to allow you to understand the problem more.

ANSWERS:

1. You have to solve the problem step by step.

    Given = C_1 = 30 mg
    V_2 = 30 ml
    C_2 = 5 mg, 10 mg, 20 mg

    Unknown = V_1

    Step #1 – Solve first the volume of the stock solution needed for each of the required concentration.

    Step #2 – Subtract the V_1 from the total volume to get volume of diluent for each required concentration.

    Step #3 – Compute for the dilution of each concentration.

    Use the formula $C_1V_1 = C_2V_2$, or ratio and proportion:

    For 5 mg:

    $C_1V_1 = C_2V_2$
    (30 mg)(V_1) = (5 mg)(30 ml)
    V_1 = [(30 ml)(5 mg)]/30 mg, or V_1 = $\underline{\text{30 ml x 5 mg}}$
     30 mg

V1 = 5 ml of stock solution

Volume of diluent = total volume - volume of stock solution
Volume of diluent = 30 ml – 5ml
Volume of diluent = 25 ml

Dilution:

Assume that the V1 value is 1 part. Thus:
5 ml = 1 part

If 1 part is 5 ml, then 25 ml = 5 parts (25/5)
1 part + 5 parts = 6 **(1:6 dilution) Answer**

For 10 mg:

$C_1V_1 = C_2V_2$
(30 mg)(V_1) = (10 mg)(30 ml)
V_1 = [(30 ml)(10 mg)]/30 mg, or V_1 = $\frac{30 \text{ ml} \times 10 \text{ mg}}{30 \text{ mg}}$

V1 = 10 ml of stock solution

Volume of diluent = total volume - volume of stock solution
Volume of diluent = 30 ml – 10ml
Volume of diluent = 20 ml

Dilution:

Assume that the value of V1 is 1 part. Thus:
10 ml = 1 part

If 1 part is 10 ml, then 20 ml = 2 parts (20/10)
1 part + 2 parts = 3 **(1:3 dilution) Answer**

For 20 mg:

$$C_1V_1 = C_2V_2$$
$$(30 \text{ mg})(V_1) = (20 \text{ mg})(30 \text{ ml})$$
$$V_1 = [(30 \text{ ml})(20 \text{ mg})]/30 \text{ mg, or } V_1 = \frac{30 \text{ ml} \times 20 \text{ mg}}{30 \text{ mg}}$$

V_1 = 20 ml of stock solution

Volume of diluent = total volume - volume of stock solution
Volume of diluent = 30 ml – 20 ml
Volume of diluent = 10 ml

Dilution:

Assume that the V_1 value is 1 part. Thus:
20 ml = 1 part

If 1 part is 20 ml, then 30 ml = 1.5 parts (30/20)
1 part + 1.5 parts = 2.5 parts **(1:2.5 dilution)**
Answer

Answers

Concentration of working solution	Volume of 30 mg stock solution	Volume of diluent	Resulting dilution
5 mg	*5 ml*	*25 ml*	*1:6*
10 mg	*10 ml*	*20 ml*	*1:3*

49

| 20 mg | *20 ml* | *10 ml* | *1:2.5* |

2. The attending physician of a 10-year old male patient has ordered that his 250-ml IV fluid must be administered within 2 hours. The drop factor of the IV burette is 15 ml per drop. What would be the correct IV flow rate?

Answer

Given:

250 ml IVF to be administered with 2 hours
Drop factor = 15 ml/drop

Unknown = IV Flow Rate

IV Flow Rate in gtt/min = $\frac{\text{Volume of fluid to be infused x drop factor}}{\text{Allotted time in minutes}}$

IV Flow Rate in gtt/min = $\frac{250 \text{ ml} \times 15 \text{ ml}}{120 \text{ minutes (2 x 60 minutes)}}$

Answer IV Flow Rate in gtt/min = 31.25 gtt.min

3. An out-patient has to take 1.5 grams (g) of erythromycin in three divided doses per day, for a

period of 1 week. If 250 mg is equal to 5 ml, how many ml will you dispense for the whole treatment?

Given:

> 1,500 mg in 3 divided doses per day for patient
> 250 mg = 5 ml

Unknown = Volume you would dispense for the whole treatment

Step #1 – Compute the total volume of erythromycin needed for the one-week treatment.

> 5.5 grams per day x 7 days (1 week) = 10.5 grams

Step #2 – Convert units to similar units.

> You can convert 10.5 grams (g) to milligrams (mg), or mg to g. But the most common unit of expression for drugs is mg.
>
> Subsequently 1 gram = 1,000 mg
>
> So, 10.5 x 1,000 = 10,500 mg for one week.

Step #3 – Compute for the total volume needed for the one week treatment.

> Using ratio and proportion of volume to weight.
>
> 250 mg/5 ml = 10,500 mg/X, or $\frac{250}{5\,ml} = \frac{10{,}500}{X}$
>
> Compute using cross multiplication and canceling out (transposing) to isolate X (unknown).

X = 10,500 x 5/250

Answer: X = 210 ml of erythromycin suspension

You will be dispensing 210 ml of erythromycin to the patient for his/her one week treatment.

4. How can you prepare a 50% solution of methanol with a total volume of 170 ml from a 95% methanol solution?

   Given:

   $C_1 = 95\%$
   $C_2 = 50\%$
   $V_2 = 170$ ml

   Unknown (X) = V_1

   You can use either ratio and proportion or $C_1V_1 = C_2V_2$
   $C_1V_1 = C_2V_2$
   $(95\%)(V_1 \text{ in ml}) = (50\%)(170 \text{ ml})$
   $V_1 = (50\%)(170 \text{ ml})/95\%$
   $V_1 = 89.47$ or 89.5 ml

   Answer: Add 89.5 ml of 95% methanol to 80.5 ml of diluent to prepare a 170 ml 50% solution.

5. A drug with an original concentration of 800 mg has been reduced to 200 mg after 90 minutes. What's the half-life of the drug?

   Given:

52

Original concentration of drug = 800 mg

Concentration after 90 minutes = 200 mg.

Unknown = half-life of drug?

Use ratio and proportion. But first determine what amount of drug was reduced by subtracting 200 mg from 800 mg.

800 mg – 200 mg = 600 mg is reduced after 90 minutes

Determine also the half-life concentration of the drug by dividing the original concentration by 2. This is because half-life is when the drug is half of its original concentration. So, 800/2 = 400 mg.

Using ratio and proportion:

600 mg:90 minutes = 400:X minutes, or $\dfrac{600 \text{ mg}}{90 \text{ min}} = \dfrac{400 \text{ mg}}{X}$

Cross multiple and transpose or cancel out the values with the unknown.

X = 400 mg x 90 minutes/600 mg

X = 60 minutes – half-life of drug

You can also solve by obtaining the amount of drug reduced per minute by dividing 600 by 90.

600/90 = 6.67 mg of drug reduced per minute

Answer: 400/6.67 = 59.97 or 60 minutes - half-life of drug

6. What dosage (in ml) would you give a patient weighing 130 pounds (lbs.) if the standard dosage is 0.1 ml per kilogram (kg) body weight?

Given:

    Weight of patient = 130 pounds
    Standard dosage = 0.1 ml per kg body weight

Unknown (X) = dosage in ml of patient weighing 130 pounds.

Again, use ratio and proportion, but you have to use similar units. You can either use kg for both units, or lbs. For this example, we will be using pounds. So, we have to convert 130 lbs. to kg by dividing the lbs. with 2.2. because 1 kg = 2.2 lbs.

Step #1 – Convert lbs. to kg.

    1kg = 2.2 lbs.; hence divide 130 lbs. by 2.2 to get the equivalent in kg.
    130/2.2 = 59.09 kg

Step #2 – Use ratio and proportion to solve main problem.

    0.1 ml:1 kg = X:59.09 kg

Take note that the volume are the numerators and the weights are the denominators. You can also make the weights, the numerators, and the volume, the denominators, provided that the values for the numerators and the denominators refer to the same aspect.

So, you can also create your ratio and proportion this way:

$$1 \text{ kg} : 0.1 \text{ ml} = 59.09 \text{ kg} : X$$

Remember that this equation can also be expressed this way:

$$\frac{1 \text{ kg}}{0.1 \text{ ml}} = \frac{59.09 \text{ kg}}{X}$$

Cross-multiply:

$$1 \text{ kg} \times X = 59.09 \text{ kg} \times 0.1 \text{ ml}$$

Transpose 59.09 kg by dividing both equations with it to solve for unknown (X):

$$X = 59.09 \text{ kg} \times 0.1 \text{ ml} / 1 \text{ kg}$$

Answer: X = 5.909 ml dosage for the person weighing 130 lbs.

7. You have performed these serial dilutions, while preparing your experimental drugs:

	Test Tube 1	Test Tube 2	Test Tube 3	Test Tube 4
	Volume in milliliters	Volume in millileters	Volume in millileters	Volume in millileters

Experimental drug /diluted drug	0.75 of pure experimental drug	0.75 from tube 1 after mixing with df	0.75 from tube 2 after mixing with df	0.75 from tube 3 after mixing with df. Discard 0.75 of the solution after mixing
Diluting fluid (df)	3	3	3	3
Final dilution	**1:5**	**1:25**	**1:125**	**1:625**

What is the final dilution of test tube no. 4?

A. 1: 25

B. 1: 625 - Answer

C. 1:3125

D. 1:125

E. 1:27

This is a serial dilution, often used in preparing solutions for experimental studies of therapeutic drugs or researches on drugs. Here are the steps in solving this problem:

Steps in computing:

Step #1 - Solve the dilutions of each tube first.

You can do this by adding the parts of the solute (experimental drug) and the solvent (diluting fluid). Keep in mind that the volume of the solute is usually considered 1 part.

Tube #1

    Volume of experimental drug or solute = 0.75 ml = 1 part
        If 1 part = 0.75 ml, then,
        3 ml of df = 4 parts (3/0.75)

Thus:

        0.75 ml of solute = 1 part
        3 ml of solvent = 4 parts
                      ----
                      5 parts

So, the dilution of tube # 1 is 1:5

Step #2 – Multiply the previous dilution to the dilution of the tube itself.

Since the contents of the tubes are the same, the dilution of the tube itself are all the same – EXCEPT for the final dilution of the 2nd and 3rd tube. You have to perform step #2.

Tube #2

    Volume of diluted experimental drug or solute = 0.75 ml = 1 part

If 1 part = 0.75 ml, then,
3 ml of df = 4 parts (3/0.75)

Thus:

0.75 ml of solute = 1 part
3 ml of solvent = 4 parts
_____
5 parts

N.B. Take note, however, that you have taken the diluted solute from tube #1, which has already been diluted. Therefore, to get the final dilution, you have to multiply the dilution of the previous tube with the dilution of the tube itself.

1:5 x 1:5 = 1:25

So, the final dilution of tube #2 is 1:25

Tube #3

Volume of diluted experimental drug or solute = 0.75 ml = 1 part
If 1 part = 0.75 ml, then,
3 ml of df = 4 parts (3/0.75)

Thus:

0.75 ml of solute = 1 part
3 ml of solvent = 4 parts
_____
5 parts

N.B. However, you have taken the diluted solute from tube #2, which has already been re-diluted. Therefore, to get the final dilution, you have to multiply the dilution of the previous tube with the dilution of the tube itself.

   1:5 x 1:25 = 1:125

So, the final dilution of tube #3 is 1:125

Tube #4

 Volume of diluted experimental drug or solute = 0.75 ml = 1 part
  If 1 part = 0.75 ml, then,
  3 ml of df = 4 parts (3/0.75)

Thus:
  0.75 ml of solute = 1 part
  3 ml of solvent = 4 parts
       ―――――
       5 parts

N.B. Take note though that you have taken the re-diluted solute from tube #3, which has already been diluted. Therefore, to get the final dilution, you have to multiply the dilution of the previous tube with the dilution of the tube itself.

   1:5 x 1:125 = 1:625

So, the final dilution of tube #4 is 1:625

8. How can you prepare a 1:10 dilution?

 A. In a test tube pipet 1 milliliter of serum and add 10 milliliters of diluent.

B. In a test tube pipet 0.5 milliliter of serum and add 4.5 milliliter of diluent.

C. In a test tube pipet 10 milliliters of serum and add 1 milliliter of diluent.

D. In a test tube pipet 0.9 milliliter of serum and add 10 milliliters of diluent.

E. In a test tube pipet 0.5 milliliter of serum and add 9.5 milliliter of diluent.

Answer: B

> Why? because as discussed earlier, the dilution is the total of the parts. If you have chosen A, it is wrong because the resulting dilution would be 1:11 (1 part + 10 parts = 11 parts (1:11 dilution).

9. What is the dilution if you have added 0.25 milliliters of serum to 2 milliliters of normal saline solution?

A. 0.25:2

B. 1:9

C. 2:0.25

D. 1:8

E. 1:2.25

Answer: B

> Because 0.25 ml = 1 part
> And 2 ml = 8 parts (if 1 part is = 0.25 ml)
>
> Add the parts: 1 part + 8 parts = 9 parts or 1:9 dilution

10. A 13-year old girl suffering from fever and myalgia was brought to the infirmary. The physician ordered 0.8 mg/kg to be injected stat. The girl weighed 120 pounds. If 1 ml is equivalent to 5 mg, how many ml would you dispense?

Step #1 – Convert weight to kg.

   120 pounds/2.2 = 54.5454545 kg

Step #2 – Multiply 0.8 mg with the weight of the girl in kg.

   0.8 x 54.55 (rounded off) = 43.64 mg

   Since 1 ml = 5 mg, 8.728 ml or **8.7 ml will be injected - Answer**

11. Express the concentration of the following substances in SI units: Use the basic SI units of measurement.

    a) 120 mg/dL glucose value = 120 x 0.0555 (c.f.)
       = **6.66 mmol/L Answer**

    b) 3 feet – Since SI units use cm, you have to convert it to cm.
       3 feet = 36 inches
       1 inch = 2.54 cm
       36 inches x 2.54 = **91.44 cm Answer**

       You can also do the previous method of cancelling out the units, if you want.

    c) 24 hours – The SI unit for time is in seconds. Hence, you have to convert hours to seconds.

61

Again, you can cancel out the units, but here's another method:

24 hours = 1440 minutes (24 x 60 because there are 60 minute in 1 hour)
1440 x 60 = 86,400 seconds (because there are 60 seconds in 1 minute

Answer: 24 hours = 86,400 seconds

12. The doctor ordered a tapering dosage of tranxene caps 5 mg, an anxiolytic drug, for a patient who has anxiety disorders. How many tranxene capsules would you dispense, if these were the orders?

    You can solve this by simply dividing the given dosage for the day by 5 and then multiplying it with the number of days. Thus:

    a) 30 mg/d. in divided doses x 3 d = 30 mg/5 mg (mg per cap) = 6 x 3 days = 18 caps of tranxene 5 mg

    b) 20 mg/d. in divided doses x 3 d = 20 mg/5 mg = 4 x 3 days = 12 tranxene caps

    c) 15 mg/d. in divided doses x 5 d = 15 mg/5 mg = 3 x 5 days = 15 tranxene caps

    d) 10mg/d x 10 d = 10 mg/5 mg = 2 x 10 days = 20 tranxene caps

    Add all the capsules for each order = 18 + 12 + 15 + 20 = 65

    Answer: 65 caps of tranxene 5 mg will be dispensed.

13. A drug is supplied in 250 mg tablets. If the prescription order is 250 mg b.i.d for a period of 10 days, how many tablets would you dispense?

    You can solve this by multiplying the frequency of the intake x the number of days.

    Tablets to be dispensed = 2 x 10 = **20 tabs** **Answer**

14. If you have dissolved 25 grams of substance in 160 ml of distilled water, what is the:
    2.1. % (W/V)
    2.2. Specific gravity

    For #2.1:

    Use the formula:

    % = W/V X 100
    % = 25 g/160 ml X 100

    Answer: % = 15.625% (W.V) solution

    For #2.2:

    Use the formula:

    Specific Gravity = Weight (density) of substance in grams
    Weight (density) of an equal volume of water in grams

Weight (density); weight = 160 ml = 160 g because the density of water is 1.

Specific Gravity = 25 g / 160 g

Answer: Sp. Gr. = 0.15625

Chapter 6: Most Significant Conversion Factors

As a pharmacist, you must be familiar with the most significant conversion factors. These conversion factors are essential when you convert the units of dosages, drugs and solutions.

Conversion factor from foot to meter = 0.3048

Example:

> All you have to do to convert 3 feet to meters is to multiply the feet with the conversion factor, which is 0.3048.
>
> 3 x 0.3048 = ***0.9144 meters (Answer)***

Conversion factor from kilograms (kg) to pounds (lbs.) = 2.2

Example:

> Convert 3.5 kg to lbs.
>
> 3.5 x 2.2 = ***7.7 lbs. (Answer)***

Conversion factor from inches to centimeters = 2.54

Example:

> Convert 12 inches to centimeters.

12 x 2.54 = ***30.48 cm (Answer)***

Based on the solution of the examples above, you can see that it's relatively easy. You just multiply the conversion factor of the value you want to convert to that unit.

Here are more conversion factors that can be helpful in converting the conventional units to SI units of the most common substances present in blood:

Substance	Conventional units	SI units	Conversion factor
BUN (Blood Urea Nitrogen)	mg% or mg/dL	mmol/L	0.357
Cholesterol	mg% or mg/dL	mmol/L	0.0258
BUA (Blood Uric Acid)	mg% or mg/dL	mmol/L	0.0595
TAG (triglyceride)	mg% or mg/dL	mmol/L	0.0113
Glucose	mg% or mg/dL	mmol/L	0.0555
Creatinine	mg% or mg/dL	umol/L	88.4
Hemoglobin	g/dL	g/L	10
Potassium	mEq/L	mmol/L	1
Calcium	mEq/L	mmol/L	0.25
Sodium	mEq/L	mmol/L	1
Chloride	mEq/L	mmol/L	1
Phosphorus (I.P.)	mEq/L	mmol/L	0.323

Basic conversions that you should know:

- 1 liter = 1,000 ml
- 1 deciliter = 100 ml
- 1 cubic centimeters (cc) = 1 ml
- 1 kilogram = 1,000 grams
- 1 gram = 1,000 milligrams (mg)
- 1 ounce = 28.35 grams
- 1 day = 24 hours
- 1 hour = 60 minutes
- 1 minute = 60 seconds
- 1 ounce = 30 ml
- 1 teaspoon = 5 ml
- 1 tablespoon = 3 teaspoons (15 ml)

You may want to learn about these most common SI prefixes, as well:

- micro (µ) = 10^{-6}
- milli (m) = 10^{-3}
- kilo (k) = 10^{3}
- mega (M) = 10^{6}
- giga (G) = 10^{9}
- tera (T) = 10^{12}

There are still several prefixes that are included, which, I hope, you have already taken up in your lectures.

Remember that this book is a reviewer and not a lecture note.

Chapter 7: Review Questions on Conversion Factors

Answer the following questions to test if you remember your conversion factors. Refrain from looking at the answers before you are done with the quiz.

Questions

1. Express the following in SI units.
   a. Cholesterol result = 230 mg/dL
   b. BUN result = 18 mgs%
   c. Creatinine = 23 mg/dL

2. The pharmacist on duty has dispensed 120 ml of cefalexin for a certain patient. If the patient is required to take 1 teaspoon t.i.d., how many days would the medication last?

3. Convert 2,575 mg to g.

4. Convert 12 dL to L.

5. Convert 21 L/20 min to ml/sec.

6. Convert 250 mg/dL to g/L.

7. Convert 10 g to kg.

8. Convert 150 ml to dL.

9. Convert 20 mmol/L to mg/dL

10. Convert 5'5" to cm.

Chapter 8: Answers to Quiz on Conversion Factors

Here are the answers to the quiz on conversion factors.

1. Express the following in SI units.
   a. Cholesterol result = 230 mg/dL
   b. BUN result = 18 mgs%
   c. Creatinine = 23 mg/dL

   Answers:

   Simply multiply the conversion factors. Keep in mind to use the SI units after conversion.

   a. Cholesterol result in SI units = 230 x 0.0258
      = ***5.934 mmol/L***

   b. BUN result in SI units = 18 x 0.357
      = ***2.294082 mmol/L***

   c. Creatinine result in SI units = 23 x 88.4
      = ***2033.2 µmol/L***

2. The pharmacist on duty has dispensed 120 ml of cefalexin for a certain patient. If the patient is required to take 1 teaspoon t.i.d. daily, how many days would the medication last?

   Given:

   120 ml – dispensed cefalexin to patient
   1 teaspoon TID – dosage of patient per day

   Unknown = days the medication will last

Step #1 – determine first how many teaspoons are there in 120 ml.

> Since 1 teaspoon = 5 ml
> So, divide 120 ml by 5 ml
> 120/5 = 24 teaspoons

Step #2 – determine how many days will the medication last

> Divide the 24 teaspoons by 3, because the patient takes 1 teaspoon of the medication 3 x per day.
> Days the medication will last = 24/3

Days the medication will last = 8

3. Convert 2,575 mg of acetaminophen to g.

   Cancel out units to solve the problem, or simply divide 2,575 mg by 1,000. This is because 1,000 mg = 1 g. Again, the ratio and proportion is also applicable in this problem. You have the choice to use the most comfortable method for you.

   Thus:

   2,575/1000 = **2.575 g acetaminophen (Answer)**

4. Convert 12 dL to L.

   Your basis is: 1 liter = 10 dL

   Thus, you can use ratio and proportion:

70

$$1\text{ L}:10\text{ dL} = X:12\text{ dL}, \text{ or } \frac{1\text{ L}}{10\text{ dL}} = \frac{X}{12\text{ dL}}$$

Cross-multiply:

$$1\text{ L} \times 12\text{ dL} = X \times 10\text{ dL}$$

Cancel out 10 dL and transpose:

$$X = \frac{1\text{ L} \times 12\text{ dL}}{10\text{ dL}}$$

Answer $X = 1.2$ L

5. Convert 21 L/20 min to ml/sec.

   You can solve this problem through cancelling out units, one by one. Start with liters first, and then followed by minutes. If the unit is in the numerator, make sure you multiply it with the unit in the denominator to cancel it out. Naturally, make use of your conversion values.

   See solution below:

   $$\frac{21\ \cancel{L}}{20\ \cancel{\text{min}}} \times \frac{1{,}000\text{ ml}}{1\ \cancel{L}} \times \frac{1\ \cancel{\text{min}}}{60\text{ sec}} = \textbf{17.5 ml/sec}$$
   (Answer)

   After cancelling out the units to convert the value to ml/sec, you can then multiply all the numerators, and then the denominators.

   You can then divide the product of the numerators by the product of the denominators.

21,000/1,200 = **17.5 ml/sec (Answer)**

You can also individually divide each fraction before multiplying. You will be obtaining the same answer.

6. Convert 250 mg/dL to g/L.

   Again, cancelling out the units you don't need until you arrive at mmol/L is the solution to this problem. Unless the substance is specified and you know the conversion factor. (See questions #1).

   $$\frac{250 \text{ mg}}{1 \text{ dL}} \times \frac{1 \text{ g}}{1{,}000 \text{ mg}} \times \frac{10 \text{ dL}}{1 \text{ L}} = \frac{2{,}500}{1{,}000}$$

   Answer: 2.5 g/L

7. Convert 10 g to kg.

   Since 1,000 g = 1 kg, you can quickly convert the value by dividing 10 g by 1,000.

   $$10 \text{ g} = 10/1000 = 0.01 \text{ kg}$$

   Answer = 0.01 kg

8. Convert 150 ml to dL.

   Since 100 ml = 1 dL, you simply divide 150 ml by 100 ml (1 dL).

   $$150 \text{ ml}/100 \text{ ml} = 1.5 \text{ dL}$$
   Answer = 1.5 dL

9. Convert 20 mmol/L of calcium to mg/dL.

   In this case, you can use the conversion factor. But instead of multiplying, you divide it, because the conversion is from SI units (mmol/L) to traditional units (mg/dL).

   The conversion factor for calcium = 0.25

   Hence:

   $$\frac{20 \text{ mmol/L}}{0.25} = 80 \text{ mg/dL}$$

   Answer = 80 mg/dL

10. Convert 5'5" to cm.

    Convert the height first to inches:

    Based on the fact that 1 foot = 12 inches, multiply 5' x 12 = 60 inches, plus 5" = 65 inches

    Next step is to multiply the inches x 2.54 to get the centimeter value. This is based on the fact that 1 inch = 2.54.

    Thus:

    $$65 \text{ inches} \times 2.54 = 165.1 \text{ cm}$$

    Answer = 165.1 cm

Chapter 9: SI Units of Measurements

The S.I. or the International System of Units is being used worldwide to standardize the units of measurement in science and the medical field.

It's also used in commerce and industry.

<u>Here are the seven base units used in SI:</u>

1. meter (m) – for length
2. second (s) – for time
3. kilogram (kg) – for weight or mass
4. mole (mol) – for amount of substance
5. ampere (A) – for electric current
6. candela (cd) – for luminous intensity
7. kelvin (K) – for thermodynamic temperature

There medical practitioners, who still use the conventional units. Most hospitals have result forms that display both the conventional and the SI units.

Nonetheless, it's best that you know the these base units, so you can convert the units on your own whenever necessary.

The SI units is recognized internationally. It's to your advantage that you learn them.

Chapter 10: Statistics in Pharmacy

In the field of pharmacy, you may encounter cases wherein you are required to compute basic statistics for drug reports, scientific studies, and for the patients' drug monitoring.

The most common statistics calculations that you may use are the following:

1. Average or arithmetic mean (X (with a bar) or Ave.)
2. Standard Deviation (SD or sd)
3. Median
4. Mode

We will discuss these 4 briefly, to review your statistics. The average or arithmetic mean:

The average, or mean is the sum of all values in a set divided by the number of values.

Example #1:

Calculate the mean of this set of values.

Concentrations of acetaminophen after half-life coming from a research respondent:

Days	Concentration of acetaminophen, after half-life
1	200 mg
2	150 mg

3	120 mg
4	180 mg
5	150 mg
Average = 160 mg	800 / 5 = 160 mg

Standard Deviation (SD or σ – sigma, the Greek alphabet)

Standard Deviation determines the dispersal or deviation of values from each other in a set. The formula for SD or σ is:

SD or σ = The square root of the sum of the difference between the mean and the individual values squared, divided by the number of values minus 1.

$$sd = \sqrt{\frac{\Sigma(\overline{X}-X)^2}{N-1}}$$

Where:

Σ = sum

$\overline{X}$ = mean or average

X = individual values

N = total number of values

Example:

Let's use the ungrouped data coming from the research study of acetaminophen from example #1.

Days	Mean $\overline{X}$	Individual values X	Difference (between mean and individual values) $\overline{X} - X$	Square of the difference $(\overline{X} - X)^2$
1	160 mg	200 mg	-40 mg	1600 mg
2	160 mg	150 mg	10 mg	100 mg
3	160 mg	120 mg	40 mg	1600 mg
4	160 mg	180 mg	-20 mg	400 mg
5	160 mg	150 mg	10 mg	100 mg
				3,800 mg

Hence:

$$\Sigma(\overline{X}-X)^2 = 3{,}800 \text{ mg}$$

You can now substitute the values in the formula:

$$sd = \sqrt{\frac{3{,}800}{5-1}}$$

Answer: sd = 30.8220700148

Pointers:

- This formula is for ungrouped data, modify your formula according to the type of data you have.
- *Steps:*
  1. Get the mean of the values
  2. Solve first for the difference between the mean and the individual values. Take note that the values are absolute, so disregard the negative signs.
  3. Square the difference between the mean and the individual values.
  4. Compute the sum of the differences between the mean and the individual values
  5. The sum from step #4 represents the entire numerator in the formula.
  6. Substitute the value you obtained from step #4 in the main formula divided by N-1.
  7. Subtract 1 from the total number of values.
  8. Solve the sd by dividing the sum of the differences with your answer to step #7 (N-1).
  9. Finally, get the square root of your answer (value) from step #8.

- Remember to square the differences between the mean and the individual values.
- Remember to compute for the square root of the final product from the division of the values.
- Keep in mind that the values are solved individually before they are substituted in the main formula.
- The higher the standard deviation, the more dispersed the values are, and the less precise. The lower the standard deviation the less dispersed the values are, but the more precise.

Median

Median is the middle value or mid-point value in a set of observed values arranged according to their magnitude.

Example #1:

concentrations of aspirin dispensed

120 mg

100 mg

80 mg

60 mg - median value

40 mg

20 mg

10mg

Example #2:

Values of glucose in SI units

2.5 mmol/L

4.5 mmol/L

6.4 mmol/L – median value

8.5 mmol/L

10.5 mmol/L

Mode

This represents the value with the most frequency in a set of values. It is the value that occurs most often among the observed values.

Example:

    Concentrations of amoxycillin

        250 mg

        120 mg

        500 mg

        250 mg

        250 mg

        500 mg

        250 mg

        120 mg

        250 mg

If you evaluate the values:

    120 mg - appeared twice (2 x)

    250 mg - appeared 5 times (5 x)

    500 mg – appeared twice (2 x)

Therefore, the mode value is 250 mg because it occurred the most in the set.

Answer =250 mg

There are still a number of statistical calculations in the field of science but let's focus on these four most common data for now.

Chapter 11: Important Medical Transcriptions and Abbreviations

As a pharmacist, you have to be familiar too with important medical transcriptions and abbreviations. Some of them may be given in the PTC exam.

There's no harm in learning the 'must know' topics. This will be an advantage for you at work, as well.

Here are the most common transcriptions, acronyms and abbreviations.

Transcriptions, acronyms and abbreviations

1. a.a. – of each
2. fl. or f - make
3. c – with
4. sig. – write or label
5. $\bar{s}$ - without
6. FBS – Fasting Blood Sugar
7. Ccr – Creatinine Clearance
8. BUA – Blood Uric Acid
9. BUN – Blood Urea Nitrogen
10. NR – No refill
11. NPO – nothing by mouth
12. TAG – triglyceride or triacylglycerol
13. ½ NS – one half normal saline or 0.45% sodium chloride solution
14. NSS – Normal Saline Solution 0.9% sodium chloride solution
15. BMI – Body Mass Index
16. C.C. – Chief Complaint
17. $\bar{c}$ – with
18. DOB – Date of Birth
19. HAART – Highly Active Antiretroviral Therapy
20. HR – Heart Rate

21. B/P – Blood Pressure
22. NSAID – Non-Steroidal Anti-Inflammatory Drug
23. OTC – Over the Counter
24. Rx – prescription
25. TPN – Total Parenteral Nutrition
26. AMS – Amylase
27. TP – Total Protein
28. BMR – Basal Metabolic Rate
29. CHS- Cholinesterase
30. LPS -Lipase

Abbreviations for measurements

$\bar{i}$ – one

ss – one half

$\bar{ss}$ – one half

tsp. – teaspoon

tbsp. – tablespoon

q.s. – sufficient quantity

q.s. ad – add ample quantity to produce

aq ad – add water up to

a.a. or aa – of each

ad – up to

ad sat – add until saturated

ml or mL – milliliter or milliliter

l or L – liter or litre

dl or dL – deciliter or deciliter

mcg. – microgram

mEq – milliequivalent

mg. – milligrams

g. or G. or gm. – grams

kg. – kilograms

lbs. – pounds

gtt. - drop

disp. – dispense

div. – divide

fl. or f – fluid

fl. oz. – fluid ounce

Abbreviations for route of administration

top. – topically

per neb – through a nebulizer

IM or i.m. – intramuscular

IV or i.v. – intravenous

IVP or i.v.p. – intravenous push

IVPB – intravenous piggyback

a.d. – right ear

a.s. or a.l. – left ear

a.u. – each ear

o.d. – right eye

o.s. or o.l. – left eye

a.u. – each eye

dil. – dilute

inj. – injection

S.L. – sublingually (under tongue)

SC, subc, subq – subcutaneously (under skin)

p.v. – through the vagina

p.r. – through rectum

p.o. – through mouth

u.d. or ut dict. – as directed

Abbreviations for time

stat – immediately

alt. – alternate

alt. h. – every other hour

o.d. – one a day

b.i.d. – twice a day

t.i.d. – thrice a day

q.i.d. – four times a day

prn – as needed

a.m. – morning

p.m. – evening, afternoon

h.s. – at bedtime

h – hour

$\bar{a}$ – before

$\bar{p}$ - after

a.c. – before meals

a.c.h.s. or achs – before meals and at bedtime

p.c. – after meals

q – every

q.d. or q1d, or QD – every day

q.o.d. – every other day

q.h. – every hour

q2h – every 2 hours

q3h – every 3 hours

q4h – every 4 hours

Abbreviations for forms of drug

amp. - ampule

liq. – liquid

elix. – elixir

cm. – cream

caps. – capsule

tabs. – tablets

oint. – ointment

syr. – syrup

sup. – suppository

aqua, aq. - water

XR, XL, SL – extended release/slow

Chapter 12: Arabic and Roman numerals

There may be questions in the PTC exam that involve Roman numerals.

A knowledge of the most commonly used items can help you pass the exam and can also broaden your knowledge of your profession.

Sometimes, doctors express the dosage - not in Arabic numerals - but in Roman numerals. Therefore, you have to know the meaning of these Roman numerals.

Most commonly used Roman numerals:

I = 1	L = 50
II = 2	LX = 60
III = 3	LXX = 70
IV = 4	LXXX = 80
V = 5	XC = 90
VI = 6	C = 100
VII = 7	CC = 200
VIII = 8	CCC = 300
IX = 9	D = 500
X = 10	M = 1,000
XX = 20	
XXX = 30	
XL = 40	

The following are essential pointers that you have to remember:

- The numerals can only be repeated thrice.
- After the third repetition, to present the next numeral, subtract by placing the numeral to be subtracted to the left of the bigger numeral, or before the next bigger value.

    Example #1:

    VIII = 8
    IX = 9
    It's not VIIII.

    Since:

    I = 1 and X = 10, hence, 10-1 = 9

    Example #2:

    XXX = 30, but XXXX is NOT 40.

    Instead, XL = 40

    Because X = 10, and L = 50

    Thus:

    50-10 = 40

- When writing your Roman numerals, use the biggest value possible. The possible numerals to subtract are only I, C and D. But not V, L, D and M.

- Keep in mind that only one lesser numeral can be placed to the left.

- More than 10-fold increase in the numeral is done differently.

- If there are numerals of lesser values that are placed after a numeral with greater value, add the amount.

- If there are numerals of lesser values that are placed before the numeral with the greater value, subtract the amount. Solve first the lesser values before adding the greater value.

Chapter 13: Review Questions on Statistics and Numerals

To evaluate if you have retained the review notes, here's a quiz about the previous three chapters.

Questions

1. 6 patients suffering from anxiety were subjected to a treatment of 5 mg of anxiolytic. Afterwards, their blood samples were tested to determine the concentration of the drug that has remained in their systems. The values are as follows:

Patients	Values obtained
1	1.2 mg
2	0.5 mg
3	0.8 mg
4	1.4 mg
5	2.0 mg
6	0.2 mg

   Determine the following:
   a) dispersal of values
   b) average

c) mode
   d) median

2. Convert the following Arabic numerals to Roman numerals:
   a) 25
   b) 36
   c) 55
   d) 58
   e) 89

3. Transcribe the following:
   a) FBS
   b) NPO
   c) d
   d) stat
   e) NSAID
   f) o.l.
   g) a.u.
   h) h.s.
   i) prn

4. The doctor wrote an order:

   Floxine fl i gtt a.u.

   What does it mean?

5. If you don't understand a medical transcription from the doctor's orders on an emergency patient, the best course of action is:
   a) Ask him directly, even if you know he may embarrass you.
   b) Make an educated guess and proceed accordingly.
   c) Research for its meaning before proceeding.
   d) Ask the nurse on duty.

e) Ask your pharmacy colleague

Chapter 14: Answers to the Review Questions

Here are the answers to the review questions on Statistics, Transcriptions and Roman Numerals.

Answers

1. 6 patients suffering from anxiety were subjected to a treatment of 5 mg of valium. Afterwards, their blood samples were tested to determine the concentration of the drug that has remained in their systems. The values are as follows:

Patients	Mean $\overline{X}$	Values obtained	$(X - \overline{X})$	$(X-\overline{X})^2$
1	1.0166667	1.2 mg	0.1833333	0.0336111
2	1.0166667	0.5 mg	0.5166667	0.2669445
3	1.0166667	0.8 mg	0.2166667	0.0469445
4	1.0166667	1.4 mg	0.3833333	0.1469444
5	1.0166667	2.0 mg	0.9833333	0.9669444
6	1.0166667	0.2 mg	0.8166667	0.6669445

				Σ (Sum) of (X − X̄)² =2.1283334

Determine the following:

a) dispersal of values – meaning the sd

Substituting the values from the computations,

$\Sigma(\overline{X}-X)^2 = 2.1283334$ mg

$$sd = \sqrt{\boxed{\frac{2.13}{6-1}}}$$

Answer: sd = 0.426

b) average

Average X̄ = sum of individual values/total number of values

= 6.1/6 = **1.0166667 Answer**

c) mode

Going over the values, all of them appeared only once.

Mode= none

d) median

Arrange the values in ascending or descending order and determine the mid-value. In this example, we will arrange the concentrations of valium in ascending order:

Values

0.2 mg
0.5 mg
0.8 mg Answer
1.2 mg
1.4 mg
2.0 mg

2. Convert the following Arabic numerals to Roman numerals:

   a) 25 = XXV
   b) 36 = XXXVI
   c) 55 = LV
   d) 58 = LVIII
   e) 89 = LXXXIX

3. Transcribe the following:

   a) FBS – Fasting Blood Sugar
   b) NPO – Nothing by mouth

c) d - day
   d) stat - immediately
   e) NSAID – Non-steroidal Anti-inflammatory Drug
   f) o.l. – left eye
   g) a.u. – each eye
   h) h.s. – at bedtime
   i) prn – as needed

4. The doctor wrote an order:

   Floxine fl 3 mg/ml
   Sig: i gtt/d a.u. x 3d

   What does it mean?

   Answer: It means you have to dispense the medicine Floxine in fluid form, and the patient has to administer 1 drop per day to each eye for 3 days.

5. If you don't understand a medical transcription from the doctor's orders on an emergency patient, the best course of action is:

   a) **Ask him directly, even if you know he may embarrass you.**
   b) Make an educated guess and proceed accordingly.
   c) Research for its meaning before proceeding.
   d) Ask the nurse on duty.
   e) Ask your pharmacy colleague

It's best to be humble, and ask directly from the person who ordered it, rather than to pretend that you know it and give the patient a medication that can be harmful to him. This could serve as a learning activity for you to learn more about your medical transcriptions.

The life of the patient is still your primary consideration.

Chapter 15: Common Drugs You Must Know

You will be dealing with drugs or medications for the rest of your career, and knowing the commonly prescribed drugs is a plus factor for you.

Don't just study for the PTC exams, but try to retain what you have learned, because it will benefit you in the long run.

1. **Salicylates** – These are acetylsalicylic drugs that are used to reduce inflammation, fever and pain. The most common example is aspirin.

    Contraindications and major side effects

    Salicylates are contraindicated in patients taking in blood thinning substances, such as warfarin. This is because they are thinning substances by themselves.

    They also interfere with platelet aggregation, thus patients with bleeding problems or blood dyscrasia must not be given the medication.

    Overdosing can cause a mixed acid-base condition because this drug can cause respiratory alkalosis and metabolic acidosis simultaneously.

    Internal hemorrhage of the small intestines can also result from drug overdose.

    It has been observed that children taking aspirin a viral infection had caused Reye's syndrome.

Reportedly, 80 mg aspirin daily has been used to prevent CVAs. This treatment, however, is still under continuous research.

2. **Acetaminophen** – This an analgesic that is safer than other types, when taken at therapeutic dosages.

   Contraindications and major side effects

   Overdosing with acetaminophen has been discovered to cause severe hepatotoxicity or hepatic necrosis. One reason is the decreased value of glutathione.

3. **Cardioactive drugs** – these are medications for cardiac conditions, such as congestive heart failure (CHF). Examples are: quinine, digoxin, disopyramide and procainamide.

   Contraindications and major side effects

   With increased dosage, atrioventricular node blockage and premature ventricular contractions (PVC) can happen.

   Also, nausea and vomiting, together with visual disturbances can occur.

4. **Antibiotics** – these are drugs that are used to treat infections. They act as antimicrobial agents.

   Examples of these are:

- aminoglycosides (tobramycin, gentamicin, amikacin) – They are usually administered through IV or IM.

Contraindications and major side effects of aminoglycosides

They should not be used with patients who have renal dysfunction. Over dosage and repeated dosages can cause nephrotoxicity, if not stopped. It can become irreversible.

It can also damage the ears, specifically the vestibular membranes and the cochlear of the inner ear.

- **Amoxicillin** (ampicillin – example, omnipen, amoxil; oxacillin – example, bactocill; penicillin – examples, ledercillin and pfizerpen)

Contraindications and major side effects of amoxicillin

It's less toxic than the other antibiotics but all drugs have side effects. It can cause diarrhea, itching, swollen tongue, bloody stool, and unusual bleeding too.

In severe overdosing, it can cause seizure, loss of consciousness, convulsions and skin rashes.

- **Tetracycline** – This drug inhibits the protein synthesis of the microorganisms, thereby inhibiting the microorganism's growth and proliferation. Examples are minocycline, achromycin V, minocin, adoxa and tetracon.

Contraindications and major side effects of tetracycline

Side effects are: burning of stomach, diarrhea and the skin's increased sensitivity to sunlight.

The drug can reduce the effectiveness of oral contraceptives and anesthetics.

- **Cephalosporin** – this drug acts as a bactericidal agent by killing bacteria directly. Examples are: keflex (cephalexin), duricef, ceclor, rocephin, and duricef.

Contraindications and major side effects of cephalosporin

The contraindication of this drug is for patients taking in medications for heartburn and acid reflux.

The side effects include, skin rashes, diarrhea, vomiting, stomachache, and oral thrush due to yeast growth.

- **Erythromycin** – this drug acts by preventing the growth and proliferation of the bacteria. Examples of this are: erythrocin,

Contraindications and major side effects of cephalosporin

The side effects are similar to that of other antibiotics. These include diarrhea, vomiting, stomach troubles, skin rashes.

One serious side effect is damage to the liver. Amber to dark yellow urine, jaundiced skin, fever and yellow discoloration of the sclera of the eye are some of the symptoms of liver disease.

The table below is a tabulated list of some common drugs together with their generic/brand names, and their general uses.

Brand Name	Generic Name	Uses
Augmentin	Amoxicillin + penicillin	Antibiotic
Lipitor®	Atorvastatin	Reduces cholesterol
Plavix®	Clopidogrel	Anti-platelet
Crestor®	Rosuvastatin	Reduces cholesterol
Glucophage	Metformin	For diabetic patients, usually Type 2 DM
Coumadin®	Warfarin	Blood thinner
Neurontin®	Gabapentin	Anti-epileptic
Valium®	Diazepam	Reduces anxiety
Deltasone®	Prednisone	Anti-inflammatory

Prozac®	Fluoxetine	Antidepressant
Purinase	Allopurinol	Anti-uric acid
Zantac®	Ranitidine	G.E.R.D
Premarin®	Estrogen	Treatment of Menopausal symptoms
Diflucan	Fluconazole	Anti-fungal
Lopressor®	Metoprolol	Hypertension, acts as beta blocker
Nexium®	Esomeprazole	G.E.R.D

There are still countless of drugs out there, but apparently, we need another book to discuss them all.

Pointers in taking therapeutic drugs:

- During medication, the entire dosage should be taken even if symptoms have subsided already. This is to ensure that the microorganism has been fully neutralized or killed.

    Stopping the medication without finishing the whole treatment course can cause the growth of drug-resistant bacteria.

- Ascertain that the patient is not allergic to the drug before taking it. Allergic reactions can become severe and could cause coma and death.

Chapter 16: Pointers in Assisting the Pharmacist in Serving Patients

In order to become a competent pharmacy technician, you will have to learn about how the procedures or processes are implemented properly.

You've come this far, congratulations!

If you feel you need a break, then by all means, do so. Relax and stretch those muscles for a while. Learning should be fun.

The first topic for this chapter is learning how to identify the components of a medication order.

Components of a medication order:

1. Date and time when the medication order was written
2. Generic or brand name of the drug
3. Route of administration of the drug
4. Dosage of the drug
5. Frequency and duration of drug treatment
6. Special orders from prescribing physician
7. If the order was written, or through telephone (T.O.), or through verbal order (V.O.), the doctor or the provider must have affixed his/her signature.
8. The licensed health practitioner taking the T.O., V.O., or written order must have signed.

All of these components must be present before you can accept and act on the medication order.

You have to assess the authenticity of the order too, and know how to identify NDC numbers correctly.

The National Drug Code (NDC)

The NDC is composed of 3-number segments: the labeler code, the product code and the package code. In the 11-digit (5-4-2) segments are followed.

In your 10-digit codes, the 3 segments can be: 4-4-2, or 5-4-1, or 5-3-2.

If you want to convert the 9-digit or 10-digit code to 11 digits, you can add a zero (0) before the appropriate segment, following the 5-4-3 format.

Examples:

5555-5555-55 (10 digits); change to 11 digits = **0**5555-5555-55

55555-555-55 (10 digits); change to 11 digits = 55555-**0**555-55

55555-5555-5 (10 digits); change to 11 digits = 55555-5555-**0**5

Notice where the zeroes (0) were inserted to make the code an 11-digit code.

The three segments of the NDC

Labeler code – FDA (Food and Drug Administration) usually assigns this first segment of the NDC (4 to 5 digits) to the manufacturer or distributor of the drug.

Product code – The labeler assigns this code. It classifies the strength or dosage form of the drug. It's usually 3 to 4 digits.

Package code – The labeler assigns this code too. It categorizes the package size and form and can be composed of 1 to 2 digits. Some manufacturers assign letters to this code, so take note of it.

Example:

55555-5555-55

Labeler code 55555 - product code 5555 - package code 55

Knowing how many digits to use will be useful when inquiring about NDC. You may eliminate the hyphens when you enter the code.

How to transfer prescriptions properly

With the use of the Internet, you can now transfer prescriptions easily to another pharmacy. However, you have to be sure that the online pharmacy is legitimate and reliable.

For the offline transfer of prescription to another licensed pharmacy, these steps can be followed:

Steps:

1. The receiving pharmacy must verify that the transferring pharmacy is licensed and that all the components of a medication order are fulfilled.

2. Records of the transfer, and signatures of persons receiving and transferring the prescription is done.

3. Aside from submitting the specified components of the medication order or prescription to the receiving pharmacy, the transferring pharmacy, must also record the following:

    o The name of the person who transferred the prescription
    o The name of the person who received the prescription
    o The name and address of the licensed pharmacy
    o The date of the transfer
    o Name and address of the patient taking the drug

4. Limitations of the transfer of prescription

    There are some limitations to this procedure that you have to be aware of. These are:

    o NR (no refill) prescriptions cannot be transferred.
    o Prescribed controlled drugs can only be transferred once.
    o If the complete dosage has been consumed, the prescription can no longer be transferred, unless a new prescription has been issued by the patient's attending physician.

Managing aseptic techniques in preparing medications and solutions

When preparing solutions and the patients' medicines, you should always apply aseptic techniques.

Microorganisms are found everywhere and on every surface around you, as you know by now.

It's imperative that you don't bring the infection to the patient through your improper methods. You can harm the patient instead of assisting in his/her therapy.

Here are proper methods to prepare medications and solutions aseptically:

Step #1 - Ensure that the preparation uses closed systems

You can use a closed-system transfer device, so that contamination coming from the environment is prevented. Likewise, it prevents the escape of fumes or vapor that can be harmful.

Also, the apparatus or materials used must be sterilized properly by a licensed manufacturer or by a reliable apparatus. This is true, if sterilization is done by the pharmacy, itself.

These materials must never be opened, until they are actually used. Aseptic needles and syringes must remain sealed. If they are exposed accidentally, they must be discarded and a new material used.

Step #2 – Ensure that all solutions are sterile and manufactured by licensed entities

The medicinal solutions or products must be sterile, and come from licensed manufacturers, who can ascertain that their products are sterile and free from infectious or contaminating substances.

Step #3 – Ensure that the pharmacist preparing the solutions or medicines has observed aseptic methods.

Constant washing or scrubbing of hands is one of the best methods to prevent the spread of microbes. In this regard, a hand-wash station must be positioned before the worker enters the controlled working area.

The person must also wear sterile gloves when working on sterile solutions and materials.

Wearing masks, gowns, and protective eyewear will not only protect the worker, but will also make sure that the solutions or medications remain sterile and are not contaminated.

The working area must be sterile and have been decontaminated. Working tables must be washed or wiped clean first with detergent and water, and then disinfected with a disinfecting agent.

Air Hepa filters (has a 99.95% air filter efficiency) and gaseous or liquid bio-decontaminators can be used to further ensure a sterile environment.

Step #4 – The person responsible must assign only 1 week as shelf-life for the solutions.

This will guarantee that solutions have remained sterile and uncontaminated.

Step #5 – Maintain an aseptically controlled environment or workplace.

The air circulating around the working area or room must contain an appropriate air-filtration system and a reliable device that can aptly maintain the sterility of the working area.

There are many devices that can help in maintaining an aseptically controlled working area, such as pharmaceutical isolator, transfer hatch, and air filters. The first two materials will operate in closed systems, where you don't need to open the material and increase the risk of contaminating it.

When your solution, medication or materials are exposed to the air or the environment, they can get contaminated.

Step #6 - *Ascertain that the pharmacist has followed the National Health Service (NHS) guidelines.* Quality assurance is required so that contamination is prevented.

Chapter 17: Inventory Control Systems

You should have a system of maintaining medications. This system will help you manage medications properly.

1. Do a regular inventory and keep track of where and when the drugs were dispensed through accurate inventories.

2. Implement a quality assurance program to test for the reliability of stored medications. You can also allow external quality assurance evaluations to determine if your pharmaceutical supplies are reliable.

3. Prevent drug theft by implementing appropriate policies and procedures.

4. Determine beforehand what pharmaceutical devices, supplies and medical equipment are needed. These must be ordered before they go out-of-stock.

5. These orders, whether these are for emergency or routine orders, have to comply with budgetary, legal, formulary and contractual policies.

6. Discard properly pharmaceutical products, devices, or supplies that are hazardous, expired, recalled, discontinued and similar types. All of these processes must be well-documented, including the name and signature of the person/s, who had performed them.

7. In cases that a change occurs, you should inform all health care professionals concerned, including the patients, of these specific changes.

8. Double check delivered products against the items that you have ordered. This is to maintain the accuracy of your inventory.

9. Prepare packages or sets of pharmaceutical supplies to facilitate dispensing or pharmacy operations.

10. Record all transactions, such as orders, received orders, removed items, discarded items and everything that has transpired in the maintenance of medications and pharmaceutical supplies. Pay attention, most especially, to how the controlled drugs and investigational products are removed or stored.

11. Set-up medication sets that can be prepared beforehand to facilitate drug dispensing.

12. Store pharmaceutical supplies properly to prevent potential hazards.

13. Ensure that pharmaceutical supplies, medicines, devices, and materials have been properly prepared, maintained, distributed and managed.

14. Set up an MSDS for the drugs, and a monitoring system to prevent errors in your inventory.

Chapter 18: System of Maintaining Medication Quality

Maintaining the quality of medications is crucial for effective treatment. The following are methods to ensure that the quality of medication is maintained.

1. A number of hospitals require that two persons sign for high-risk medications. This will ascertain that the medication is properly dispensed to the right patient.

2. Safe systems of patient care have to be developed and observed by the health institution.

3. The handling and maintenance of the medications must comply with existing policies of the community created for that purpose.

4. Standard Operational Procedures (SOPs) have to be created to respond to all aspects of the process. This must be in detail, clear and has been disseminated accurately to all health care workers.

5. The SOPs have to be in compliance with existing federal and institutional laws and policies.

6. The health professionals handling the medications must have appropriate training.

7. Medications have to be labelled and handled properly, with a system that can systematically address accidents and errors in handling the therapeutic medications.

8. Health personnel that has to administer medicines intravenously or intramuscularly must observe aseptic methods to avoid contamination of the medicine.

9. Proper precautions must also be in place so that the preparation of the medications will not be compromised.

10. Transferring medications may affect their quality, if correct procedures are not implemented. The transfer of the drugs must be duly authorized, and also recorded properly with the name and signature of persons sending and receiving it. The date of transfer, the name of the drug and the patient must also be specified.

    Use tamper-evident and secure containers to transport the medicines. The staff must also be properly trained on how to maintain the integrity of the drugs.

11. The medicines have to be secured properly to avoid tampering or loss. Being careless with them could cause contamination with infective agents or impurities.

12. There should be an SOP on the correct storage, handling and preparation of the drugs or medications, and a Material Safety Data Sheet (MSDS) ready in cases of emergencies. The MSDS will provide information on the toxic effects of all harmful substances, and the appropriate steps on how to cope with in cases of accidents.

    The pharmacy's SOP has to be approved, documented, and disseminated properly. This should cover hazardous incidents and accidents related to the medications.

In summary, you have to maintain the quality of your medication by setting up checks and balances to ensure that the integrity of the drugs is maintained.

Pharmacy Billing and Reimbursement

The pharmacy is responsible in billing the patient's insurance company for the medications. You must fill out the forms accurately to avoid errors, which can be costly.

In the procurement stage, the drug obtained is converted to UOM, the storage units of measure. The data must be uploaded correctly to avoid errors.

The UOMs must be reconciled properly to avoid over or under charging the patient. There must also be a monitoring system that can quickly detect inconsistencies. Most hospitals are now automated, so you can perform billing and reimbursement smoothly.

Chapter 19: Administration and Management of Pharmacy Practice

Pharmacy practice encompasses various aspects of this profession. It's a rewarding career and a commendable way to develop your sense of responsibility and dedication.

Pharmacy Operations

There are three major resources that can affect the successful operations of a pharmacy. These are capital, materials or devices, and human resources or people. The third one is the most important. Without reliable and competent employees, success can never be attained.

Without human resources, the health institution cannot achieve its set objectives. This goes true with pharmacy operations. The goal must be to provide reliable and efficient health care services through the integration of relevant and applicable methods.

How to maintain pharmacy equipment

The equipment used have to calibrated and monitored regularly. Inaccurate equipment can cause errors in the preparation of medications.

Each equipment has a calibrating period. You have to be aware of this. Keep in mind that the use of updated and state of the art devices, such as automation, is a requirement, if you want your pharmacy operations to flow smoothly.

How to keep records

Keeping records is vital in the administration and management of a pharmacy practice.

It has been previously discussed that all procedures and processes have to be well-documented. It's only through documentation that you can easily trace the sources of errors, the pharmacy operations, and the acquisition and dispensing of drugs.

Managing controlled drugs

As a pharmacist or pharmacy technician, one of your responsibilities is to handle controlled drugs. Here are vital steps that you must do:

Step #1 – Be aware of currently existing legislative laws and SOPs.

In handling controlled drugs, you should follow any existing legislative or federal laws for the drugs. In addition, you must also comply with current SOPs, which are in place. Do some research to keep abreast of both these primary considerations.

Don't rely on what you already know because there may be modifications or changes in the practice that you are not aware of. Thus, confirm what is required from both before you take action.

Step #2 – Document the movement of the controlled drug at the onset.

The designated person receiving the controlled drug has to double check thoroughly, if the received items are the same items requested. The person in charge should carefully inspect the delivery, if the name, quantity, drug form, and similar aspects are as ordered previously. That's why keeping a record of the requisition slip is also important.

Step #3 – The receipt of the controlled drug must be documented using controlled drugs register.

Record the receipt of the controlled drug, documenting the date and time the drug was received; by whom; the nature, name, quantity, form and other pertinent aspects of the controlled drug.

This indicates that each department should have its own controlled drugs register. This is where all transactions about the controlled drug in that particular department are recorded.

Step #4 – Store the controlled drug in accordance to the Controlled Substances Act (CSA) and the FDA.

The CSA and the FDA have rules on controlled drugs that you have to comply with. It's common sense that you must also follow good practices in pharmacy to store your drugs.

The arrangement of the drugs when stored should follow the safety storage regulations

Step #5 - Secure the controlled drugs safely to prevent theft and loss.

If the amount of the controlled drugs is large, you can seek the assistance of concerned authorities, such as security or crime prevention officers to ensure that the drugs are safe and secure.

The controlled drugs must be secured 24/7 by designated health personnel or assigned security officers. The pharmacy staff have to supervise the storage of the drug 24/7

Step #6 – The controlled drugs must be audited regularly

If the audit cannot be done daily, or weekly, or monthly, at least the ensure that every 3 months auditing or inventory is done to reconcile your stock balance. This is an important step because the personnel in-charge may be re-assigned or may resign. In this case, the records would still be intact and easy to use in monitoring the controlled drugs. DEA has imposed a biennial inventory of the controlled drugs.

Step #7 – Dispose the unused controlled drug properly.

Before disposing any of the controlled drugs, this procedure must be documented in the controlled drugs register. The persons involved in each step of the disposal must be noted and recorded. The senior pharmacist is usually in-charge in disposing them, or he/she may at least be present.

The disposal of controlled drugs that were prepared for a particular patient but were not consumed when in the ward must be destroyed in the presence of a witness, an authorized health personnel.

In cases, when the shelf-life of the controlled drug has expired, it can be returned for destruction.

Any destruction of the controlled drugs must follow the Special Waste Policy guidelines, and must be witnessed by designated authorities.

Remember that controlled drugs are harmful and dangerous, so proper precautions in handling them must be observed.

Chapter 20: Responsibilities of a Pharmacy Technician to Patients

Apart from the apparent responsibility of a pharmacist or pharmacy technician of preparing and providing medications for patients, there are additional tasks that you have to do.

Observing confidentiality

Like any other medical professional, you must observe confidentiality regarding your patient's personal information. The patient's personal information is protected under the edict of Professional Secrecy.

It's the right of the patient to have his personal information protected from other people, and it's the responsibility of the pharmacy office and other related health departments to observe this principle of Professional Secrecy.

This means you cannot reveal any information about the patient unless the patient has authorized it, or has given his consent verbally or in writing. In cases when the patient cannot do so, only close family members (parents and siblings) may have access to his condition and personal records.

Only medical professionals involved in the treatment of the patient must be informed of the patient's condition.

Methods to maintain Professional Secrecy

- During consultation, use a private area where people cannot overhear your conversation.
- Health professionals must discuss patients' cases in private.

- Never release any information online or through phone, if you're unsure if the person is authorized or not.

Some of the patient's personal information that have to be protected are:

- Medical history
- Allergies
- Past and present illnesses
- Demographic information and other info (name, age, gender, address, credit cards and similar information)
- Medications
- Surgical procedures undertaken

Your patients trust you, so you must not betray that trust by being careful of accidentally or purposely revealing any of their personal information.

How to Handle Drug Recalls

There can be instances when you have to handle Drug Recalls. Usually, drugs are recalled by the manufacturer of the drug itself, or the hospital, or authorized agencies (FDA). The Drug Recall is done when drugs have been observed to be mislabeled, contaminated, or dangerous by

When these happens, here are steps you can implement:

Step #1 - The head of the pharmacy and designated health officers must be informed.

All personnel must be informed of the Drug Recall, the pharmacy, the medical and the nursing staff. The head of the pharmacy must act promptly to prevent further dispensation of the drug.

Step #2 - Retrieve the drugs

If you're the head pharmacist, you have to retrieve the drugs from all areas of the hospital where it has been distributed (dispensing areas, pharmacy, ER, pharmacy store room). All drugs in the storage area must be removed immediately to prevent its availability.

In-patients taking the drug must discontinue immediately and return them. The pharmacy staff must do the rounds to confirm that all drugs are recalled from in-patients.

Step #3 – Inform prescribers and other support groups

The prescribers and their support groups must be informed of the Drug Recall, so they can discontinue instantly and stop prescribing the drug.

Step #4 – Prescriptions of out-patients must be recalled and discontinued

They must be informed of the danger of their continued use of the drug. Their questions must be aptly addressed to let them understand the reason.

Step #5 – All the drugs recalled are returned

The recalled drugs must be labeled 'RECALLED' to ascertain that no one uses them. They can be returned to the manufacturer or to the recalling agency, or government entity.

If they are stored in the pharmacy storage room, they must be labeled 'RECALLED' and the following data noted: brand name, generic name, lot number, date of manufacture, expiration date, and quantity of the drug. This report must be signed by a designated hospital personnel.

Step #6 – Record all information about the recalled drugs

Make sure you have documented all information about the recalled drugs. This should include: names or patients, names of personnel who returned the drug, place from where the drug came from, quantity of the drug, date and time returned, code number of the drug (if any), condition of the drug, type of drug, and other pertinent information.

A copy of the record should be left in the pharmacy office for future reference.

Step #7 – Determine the severity of the 'RECALL'

You can do this by using this basis:

> *Class I* – The recalled drug can cause irreversible and permanent adverse side effects.
>
> *Class II* – The adverse side effects are temporary, reversible and non-life threatening.
>
> *Class III* – There are no known adverse side effects of the drugs.

Whatever the severity of the DRUG RECALL, all concerned entities must be informed of the status of the recall.

Chapter 21: Review Questions for the PTC Exams

The review questions cover all topics included in the PTC exams. Therefore, you will have to use all the information you have already learned not only from this review book, but from all other resources.

Understandably, not all of the topics are presented in this book because the primary purpose of this book is to REVIEW you, and not to conduct in-depth lectures. This activity should be done in a regular lecture setting.

Nevertheless, the correct answers are discussed to further increase your chances of passing the PTC exams.

Refrain from looking at your notes when answering the questions. You should only peruse your notes, after you have finalized your answers.

Try to allot yourself 1 minute to answer each question. This will train you for the actual exams. You can always re-take the exam in this book, whenever you want.

The questions in the PTC exam are multiple-type questions, but some questions that requires you to answer in essay form are included to hone your analytical skills. This can help you later on when you will be taking the actual test.

Instructions:

Answer the questions as specified. For multiple-type questions, choose the BEST ANSWER.

<u>Questions</u>

1. The following are observed in the disposal of controlled drugs, EXCEPT:

a) Before disposing any of the controlled drugs, the procedure must be documented in the controlled drugs register.
b) The persons involved in each step of the disposal must be noted and recorded.
c) The senior pharmacist is usually in-charge in disposing controlled drugs.
d) Controlled drug medications not administered to the patient, when in the ward, must be given to the patient because it belongs to him.
e) The correct disposal of controlled drugs that have expired shelf-life is to return them to the designated authority for destruction.

2. The doctor has written the prescription for his patient (see image below): Based on this, answer the following questions.

   a) What is the drug prescribed?
   b) What's the dosage of the medicine?
   c) Is there something wrong with the prescription? Specify and correct the errors, if any.
   d) How many tablets would the patient need for the total prescribed set?
   e) What's the purpose of the prescribed drug?

Richard N. Mill, MD

120 Reed Avenue

San Diego, California, 92093

Tel. (619) 365-6154 Fax. (619) 321-5327

Name: <u>Vanessa Park</u> Date: <u>January 1, 2018</u>

Address: <u>San Diego, California</u>

XX

:

<u>Richard N. Mill, MD</u>

CA 246810

metropolol 5 mg
x

Sig 1 tab bid x 7d

3. How would a prescription for patient, Bill Snowden from Idaho be filled out? The medication is amikacin 500 mg ampule to be injected intravenously twice a day, for 1 week. Write down the prescription.

4. The stock balance of the controlled drug must be reconciled at least every three months:

    a) To monitor the disposal of the controlled drug, internally and externally
    b) To check if the controlled drug received, dispensed and stocked are all accounted for
    c) To determine if the shelf-life of the drug has expired
    d) To assess the situation of the controlled drug for quality assurance purposes
    e) To ensure that the controlled drug has undergone proper documentation

5. Health personnel that has to administer medicines intravenously or intramuscularly must observe the following steps, EXCEPT:

    a) Observe aseptic methods to avoid contamination of the medicine and the materials used
    b) Use sterile materials to prevent infecting the patient
    c) Prevent unnecessary exposure of the medicine to air because the air may contain pathogens harmful to the patient
    d) Prepare materials properly by opening the syringe pack and testing it before administration
    e) Wash hands properly

6. The Controlled Substances Act, which specifies that the stock balance of controlled drugs must be reconciled biennially is implemented by:
    a) American Medical Association (AMA)
    b) Pharmacy Formulary Committee (PFC)

c) Drug Enforcement Administration (DEA)
   d) Hospital Pharmacist Association (HPhA)
   e) World Health Organization (WHO)

7. A 22-year old woman complaining of tenesmus and diarrhea was diagnosed with amoebiasis. The physician has prescribed Metronidazole 1,500 mg in 3 divided doses per day, for 10 days. What would you dispense?
   a) 30 tabs of flagyl 500 mg
   b) 60 caps of aralen 250 mg
   c) 60 tabs of pyrantel 250 mg
   d) 150 tabs of metrifonate 100 mg
   e) 30 caps of cloxacillin 500 mg

8. A 60-year old man collapsed on the street and was rushed to the ER of the hospital you're working in. The vital signs taken were: PR = 100 bpm, B/P = 180/110; T = 36.8 degrees C; RR = 29 breaths per minute. What medication would the doctor most probably request stat?
   a) Captopril 25 mg sl taken sublingually
   b) Amidotrizoate 140 mg amp. injected intramuscularly
   c) Furosemide 40 mg tab taken orally
   d) Hydrocortisone 100 mg vial injected intravenously
   e) Vibramycin 100 mg taken orally

9. There are various routes of drug administration to patients. The most common and most convenient method for majority of patients is this method:
   a) IV
   b) IM
   c) Oral
   d) Rectal
   e) subc

10. The Material Safety Data Sheet (MSDS) is vital to pharmacy operations while in the workspace because:

a) It provides the complete list of materials and equipment and how to operate them safely
b) It records the inventory of all materials used in pharmacy operations
c) It provides information on the harmful effects of substances and how to deal with them
d) It is a compilation of all the safety SOPs of the hospital
e) It is a data sheet that is used in ensuring the patients' safety

11. If you went on a drinking spree, what therapeutic drug must you avoid to prevent exacerbation of the side effects of alcohol?
    a) Dimetapp tabs
    b) Betaloc tabs
    c) Diatabs tabs
    d) Gentamicin injection
    e) Zovirax cream

12. When a harmful substance is spilled on your workplace table, the proper thing to do is to:
    a) Wipe the spilled substance immediately using disposable gloves and rags
    b) Refer to the substance's MSDS to follow the instructions
    c) Inform the chief pharmacist and ask what to do
    d) Spray it with a sterilizing agent and clean it afterwards
    e) Wear protective gear and wash the table thoroughly with soap and water

13. The doctor has prescribed 10 mg Zocor 10 mg tabs b.i.d./day for 30 days to a patient suffering from atherosclerosis. You are tasked to dispense and receive payment for the purchase of the medication. The Zocor 10 mg is $5.25 per tab, while the Zocor 20 mg is $9.60. The patient is in a financial bind, and he requested that

he be allowed to buy the 20 mg instead, because it's cheaper. How many Zocor 20 mg would you dispense, and how much was he able to save?
a) 60 tabs of Zocor 20 mg; $30
b) 30 tabs of Zocor 20 mg; $27
c) 15 tabs of Zocor 20 mg; $15
d) 60 tabs of Zocor 20 mg; $40
e) 30 tabs of Zocor 20 mg; $18

14. The following drugs are calcium channel blockers, EXCEPT:
a) Norvasc
b) Adalat
c) Cardizem
d) Procardia
e) Cordarone

15. The fasted route of administration of drugs to the human body is:
a) Orally
b) Intramuscularly
c) Intravenously
d) Rectally
e) Subcutaneously

16. The most common cause of emergency cases in children due to overdosing is:
a) Paracetamol
b) Aspirin
c) Erythromycin
d) Plavix
e) Cefalexin

17. The recommended temperature in storing drugs, which require refrigeration is:
a) 0°C
b) 8°C
c) 15°F

d) 4°C
   e) 30°F

18. The major organ responsible in the detoxification and breakdown of drugs taken in by a person is the:
    a) Liver
    b) Kidney
    c) Stomach
    d) Small intestines
    e) Pancreas

19. The concentration of the drug that is most beneficial to the patient is the:
    a) Sub-therapeutic concentration
    b) Toxic concentration
    c) Maximum concentration
    d) Therapeutic concentration
    e) Optimum concentration

20. Aseptic techniques in pharmacy is critical to ensure that medications, devices, and solutions remain sterile. The following are methods to ensure this, EXCEPT:
    a) Use Hepa air filters to filter out 99.955 of microbes.
    b) As much as possible, use a closed system, wherein human intervention is minimized.
    c) Sterile protective gear such as gloves, gown, masks must be worn in the preparation room,
    d) Disposable materials used in preparing medications must be autoclaved properly
    e) Only chemically pure reagent grade substances must be used in preparing working solutions

Chapter 22: Answers to Review Questions on PTC Exams

Here are the answers to the review questions. The answers are in blocked letters. The original question is included to provide clarity, and to increase retention. An explanation is given after each question.

1. The following are observed in the disposal of controlled drugs, EXCEPT:

    a) Before disposing any of the controlled drugs, the procedure must be documented in the controlled drugs register.
    b) The persons involved in each step of the disposal must be noted and recorded.
    c) The senior pharmacist is usually in-charge in disposing controlled drugs.
    d) **Controlled drug medications not administered to the patient, when in the ward, must be given to the patient because it belongs to him.**
    e) The correct disposal of controlled drugs that have expired shelf-life is to return them to the designated authority for destruction.

    Answer: d

    As discussed earlier, the controlled drug prepared but not administered to the patient must not be given to the patient, but must be destroyed right there in the ward, in the presence of a second authorized health professional.

2. The doctor has written the prescription for his patient (see image below): Based on this, answer the following questions.

   Answers:

   a) What is the drug prescribed? - ***Metoprolol 5 mg***
   b) What's the dosage of the medicine? – ***1 tablet twice a day***
   c) Is there something wrong with the prescription? Specify and correct the errors, if any.

   - ***The Rx symbol is missing. Although it's understood that the piece of paper is a medical prescription, it's still best to add the Rx symbol to avoid ambiguities.***

   - ***The number of prescribed metoprolol (XXX= 30) is not the same as the required dosage (2 tabs x 7 days = 14). The actual number of needed tablets is only 14 and not 30. However, since metoprolol is usually a maintenance drug, the excess prescribe number can be carried over to the succeeding days after the 7 days. But, you should confirm this first with the patient's attending physician.***

   d) How many tablets would the patient actually need for the total prescribed set?

   2 tabs x 7 days = ***14 tabs of metoprolol***

   e) What's the purpose of the prescribed drug?

It's a beta blocker, lowering the B/P of hypertensive patients.

Richard N. Mill, MD

120 Reed Avenue

San Diego, California, 92093

Tel. (619) 365-6154 Fax. (619) 321-5327

Name: <u>Vanessa Park</u> Date: <u>January 1, 2018</u>

Address: <u>San Diego, California</u>

xx

:

<u>Richard N. Mill, MD</u>

CA 246810

metoprolol 5 mg
×

Sig 1 tab bid × 7d

3. How would a prescription for patient, Bill Snowden from Idaho be filled out? The medication is amikacin 500 mg ampule to be injected intravenously twice a day, for 1 week. Write down the prescription.

Answer is found below.

Richard N. Mill, MD

120 Reed Avenue

San Diego, California, 92093

Tel. (619) 365-6154 Fax. (619) 321-5327

Name: <u>Bill Snowden</u>   Date: <u>May 5, 2017</u>

Address: <u>Idaho</u>

Rx:

    Amikacin 500 mg amp

Sig: 1 amp IV b.i.d. x 7 d

<u>Richard N. Mill, MD</u>
CA 246810

Of course, the prescription must be written by hand.

4. The stock balance of the controlled drug must be reconciled at least every three months:

   a) To monitor the disposal of the controlled drug, internally and externally
   b) ***To check if the controlled drug received, dispensed and stocked are all accounted for***

c) To determine if the shelf-life of the drug has expired
d) To assess the situation of the controlled drug for quality assurance purposes
e) To ensure that the controlled drug has undergone proper documentation

Answer: b

All of the other choices can be the reason for performing the inventory, but letter b is the BEST ANSWER because that's the primary purpose of the inventory.

5. Health personnel that has to administer medicines intravenously or intramuscularly must observe the following steps, EXCEPT:

a) Observe aseptic methods to avoid contamination of the medicine and the materials used
b) Use sterile materials to prevent infecting the patient
c) Prevent unnecessary exposure of the medicine to air because the air may contain pathogens harmful to the patient
d) Prepare materials properly by opening the syringe pack and testing it before administration
e) Wash hands properly

Answer: d

You should never open your syringe pack, if you're not ready to use. You can easily check it before the procedure. Opening the pack prematurely can increase the risk of contamination.

6. The Controlled Substances Act, which specifies that the stock balance of controlled drugs must be reconciled biennially is implemented by:
   a) American Medical Association (AMA)
   b) Pharmacy Formulary Committee (PFC)
   c) ***Drug Enforcement Administration (DEA)***
   d) Hospital Pharmacist Association (HPhA)
   e) World Health Organization (WHO)

   Answer: c

   The DEA is responsible in implementing the CSA.

7. A 22-year old woman complaining of tenesmus and diarrhea was diagnosed with amoebiasis. The physician has prescribed Metronidazole 1,500 mg in 3 divided doses per day, for 10 days. What would you dispense?
   a) ***30 tabs of flagyl 500 mg***
   b) 60 caps of aralen 250 mg
   c) 60 tabs of pyrantel 250 mg
   d) 150 tabs of metrifonate 100 mg
   e) 30 caps of cloxacillin 500 mg

   Answer: a

   To determine the number of 500 mg flagyl, divide 1,500 by 500. This will give you 3.

   Then multiply 3 x 10 = to get the number of tabs to be dispensed.

   3 x 10 = 30 tablets

8. A 60-year old man collapsed on the street and was rushed to the ER of the hospital you're working in. The vital signs taken were: PR = 100 bpm, B/P = 180/110; T = 36.8 degrees C; RR = 29 breaths per minute. What

medication would the doctor most probably request stat?
- **a) *Captopril 25 mg sl taken sublingually***
- b) Amidotrizoate 140 mg amp. injected intramuscularly
- c) Furosemide 40 mg tab taken orally
- d) Hydrocortisone 100 mg vial injected intravenously
- e) Vibramycin 100 mg taken orally

Answer: a

Captopril is an anti-hypertensive drug, and the rest of the choices are not. Amidotrizoate is for constipation; Furosemide is a diuretic used in reducing edema in CHF (Congestive Heart Failure); hydrocortisone is a steroid used in treating inflammations and some skin diseases; and vibramycin is an antibiotic belonging to the tetracycline family.

Based on the patient's findings, he has hypertension based on his 180/110 B/P. The normal B/P for his age is usually 120/80.

His RR (respiration rate) and PR (pulse rate) are slightly elevated but this is apparently physiological because of hypertension.

Normal RR at rest – 12 to 20 breaths per minute
Normal PR at rest – 60 to 100 bpm

9. There are various routes of drug administration to patients. The most common and most convenient method for majority of patients is this method:
   - a) IV
   - b) IM
   - **c) *Oral***
   - d) Rectal

e) subc

Answer: c

This is because the oral route is non-invasive and is easily performed. On the other hand, all the other methods are invasive. They can inflict pain on the patient. Unless the health worker is an expert, the IM, IV and subc routes can hurt the patient. The rectal method is inconvenient and least popular.

10. The Material Safety Data Sheet (MSDS) is vital to pharmacy operations, while in the workspace because:
    a) It provides the complete list of materials and equipment and how to operate them safely
    b) It records the inventory of all materials used in pharmacy operations
    c) It provides information on the harmful effects of substances and how to deal with them
    d) It is a compilation of all the safety SOPs of the hospital
    e) It is a data sheet that is used in ensuring the patients' safety

    Answer: c

    Each substance must have an MSDS, so that anyone can quickly be provided with information about the substance and how to deal with issues arising from it.

11. If you went on a drinking spree, what therapeutic drug must you avoid to prevent exacerbation of the side effects of alcohol?
    a) Dimetapp tabs
    b) Betaloc tabs

c) Diatabs tabs
d) Gentamicin injection
e) Zovirax cream

Answer: a

Dimetapp is a decongestant and an antihistamine, which can exacerbate the effects of alcohol, such as drowsiness, CNS depression, and similar symptoms.

12. When a harmful substance is spilled on your workplace table, the proper thing to do is to:
    a) Wipe the spilled substance immediately using disposable gloves and rags
    b) Refer to the substance's MSDS to follow the specified instructions
    c) Inform the chief pharmacist and ask what to do
    d) Spray it with a sterilizing agent and clean it afterwards
    e) Wear protective gear and wash the table thoroughly with soap and water

    Answer: b

    Wiping the spilled substance without knowledge of the dangers that it may pose, is irresponsible.

    You can inform the chief pharmacist later on, if you cannot resolve the issue.

    If you spray the substance with a sterilizing agent, the agent may react with the substance that may cause more accidents.

    Wearing a protective gear without knowing what the substance can do is pointless. The substance may be corrosive and your protective gear will only increase your risk of being harmed.

13. The doctor has prescribed 10 mg Zocor 10 mg tabs b.i.d./day for 30 days to a patient suffering from atherosclerosis. You are tasked to dispense and receive payment for the purchase of the medication. The Zocor 10 mg is $5.25 per tab, while the Zocor 20 mg is $9.60. The patient is in a financial bind, and he requested that you allow him to buy the 20 mg tabs instead because it's cheaper. How many Zocor 20 mg would you dispense, and how much was he able to save?
    a) 60 tabs of Zocor 20 mg; $30
    b) 30 tabs of Zocor 20 mg; $27
    c) 15 tabs of Zocor 20 mg; $15
    d) 60 tabs of Zocor 20 mg; $40
    e) 30 tabs of Zocor 20 mg; $18

    Answer: b
    Step #1 – Determine how much Zocor 20 mg will the patient need.

    Since the patient only needs 10 mg per dose, one 20 mg is sufficient for the day. So, in one day, only 1 tab of Zocor 20 mg is needed.

    Step #2 – Solve how many Zocor 20 mg does the patient need.

    1 (no. of Zocor needed for a day) x 30 (no. of days) = 30 Zocor 20 mg tabs is needed by the patient.

    Step #3 – Compute the difference of the prices.

    Compute now for the difference in the prices of the 10 mg and 20 mg.

Since the patient needs 20 mg per day, if the patient purchases the 10 mg, he has to buy two tabs.

10 mg (2 tabs) = $5.25 x 2 = $10.50

20 mg (1 tab) = $9.60

Compute the difference between the prices of the 10 and 20 mg to obtain the amount saved.

$10.50 - $9.60 = $0.90 amount saved per day

Since the medication will last a month, multiply the daily savings with 30 days.

$0.90 x 30 days = $27.00

Answer: With 30 tabs of Zocor 20 mg purchased, the patient can save $27.00 in a month

14. The following drugs are calcium channel blockers, EXCEPT:
    a) Norvasc
    b) Adalat
    c) Cardizem
    d) Procardia
    e) Cordarone

   Answer: e

Cordarone is an antiarrhythmic drug and a cardio glycoside, while the rest of the choices are all calcium blockers.

149

15. The fastest route of administration of drugs to the human body is:
    a) Orally
    b) Intramuscularly
    c) Intravenously
    d) Rectally
    e) Subcutaneously

    Answer: c

    The IV and sublingual routes are the fastest because in the IV route, the drug can be transported directly through the blood to the site of action. The second is sublingual. The various capillaries under the tongue can transport the drug to the bloodstream swiftly, without passing through the digestive system.

    Passing through the digestive system will lengthen the process because the drug has to undergo the full process.

    Before the medication or drug can act, it must be transported first to the area where it's needed. The means of transportation in the body is through the bloodstream. So, in the other route of administration, the time for the drug to act is longer because the drug has to reach the bloodstream first.

    The slowest route is the rectal method. This is only used when there is no other way of administering the drug.

    In the pharmacokinetics of drugs, the processes that occur inside the body are the ADME: Absorption, Distribution, Metabolism and Elimination.

    First the drug is absorbed in the body and then distributed to the other parts of the body.

Metabolism occurs in the liver, where the drug is detoxified and converted into a lesser toxic substance.

Afterwards, the drug goes to the site of action and will be eventually eliminated. The route of elimination are the pores of the skin, the kidneys (urine), the liver, the lungs and the digestive system (stool).

16. The most common cause of emergency cases in children due to overdosing is:
    a) Paracetamol
    b) Aspirin
    c) Erythromycin
    d) Plavix
    e) Cefalexin

    Answer: b

    Aspirin or salicylate is the most common cause of emergency toxicology in children. This is due to the sweet taste and colorful presentation of the drug (aspilets).

    Keep the medicine in a safe and secure place where the child cannot reach it. Don't let the drug be scattered carelessly inside the house.

    Reportedly, the overdosing usually occurred due to misplaced aspirin tablets.

17. The recommended temperature in storing drugs, which require refrigeration is:
    a) 0°C

b) 8°C
c) 15°F
d) 4°C
e) 30°F

Answer: d

This is the temperature that most medical supplies require. Read the labels though, to confirm that you are storing the drug correctly. For longer storage, freezing may be required.

18. The major organ responsible in the detoxification and breakdown of drugs taken in by a person is the:
    a) Liver
    b) Kidney
    c) Stomach
    d) Small intestines
    e) Pancreas

    Answer: a

    The liver is the major metabolic organ of the body. It is also where some enzymes interact with the drug. The liver detoxifies most drugs that passes through it. That's why it's also called the 'first-pass-route'.

19. The concentration of the drug that is most beneficial to the patient is the:
    a) Sub-therapeutic concentration
    b) Toxic concentration
    c) Maximum concentration
    d) Therapeutic concentration
    e) Optimum concentration

    Answer: d

In Therapeutic Drug Monitoring (TDM), the sub-therapeutic concentration is the concentration of the drug that does not have any action on the infective agent.

The toxic concentration is the amount of drug that is fatal or harmful to the patient.

The therapeutic concentration is the amount of drug that can cure the illness.

This is the main purpose of TDM: to establish the therapeutic range for patients. Treatment can then be individualized according to the various factors in the patient's body.

The factors are:

a) The patient's liver and kidney function
b) The rout of administration
c) The concentration of the drug taken
d) The metabolism of the drug in the body
e) The pharmacokinetics of the drug inside the patient's body
f) The pharmacodynamics of the drug inside the patient's

20. Aseptic techniques in pharmacy is critical to ensure that medications, devices, and solutions remain sterile. The following are methods to ensure this, EXCEPT:
a) Use Hepa air filters to filter out 99.955 of microbes.
b) As much as possible, use a closed system, wherein human intervention is minimized.
c) Sterile protective gear such as gloves, gown, masks must be worn in the preparation room,

d) Disposable materials used in preparing medications must be autoclaved properly
e) Only chemically pure reagent grade substances must be used in preparing working solutions

Answer: d

The question has the word "EXCEPT", hence the answer is d, because all of the other choices are correct, except d. Disposable materials are NOT reusable. They should never be autoclaved or sterilized for a second use.

Instead, they should be discarded properly, in a manner that they will not contaminate other people.

Conclusion

The future is bright for you. You have taken the first step in ensuring that you pass the PTC exams. Now all you need is to focus on your quest.

With the correct attitude and the determination to learn, you have increased your chances of passing the test.

Continue reviewing and you will surely achieve success in the long run. Go for it!

CPSIA information can be obtained
at www.ICGtesting.com
Printed in the USA
FSHW020715251020
75213FS